# Keto Cookbook
# for Women
# Over 50

The Ultimate and Complete Ketogenic Diet
Guide for Senior Beginners After 50 with 150
Weight Loss Keto Recipes (including
Vegetarian), 30 Days Meal Plan, Shopping List
and Tips for Healthy Eating Away from Home

**Dr. Suzanne Ramos Hughes, Amy Ryan**

## Legal & Disclaimer

# Table of Contents

# INTRODUCTION

Life after you turn fifty is quite different. Your body suddenly starts experiencing behaviors that start off as weird. They are inconvenient but after a while, you accept them and throw them under the 'I'm getting old' table. However, that is not always the case. Some of these negative symptoms are actually a result of our habits.

At 50, it is more important than ever that you eat more healthy foods. Unlike decades earlier, you cannot get away with careless and unplanned meals; each calorie and carb matters. When you eat healthily, you not only gain health, but you also lose weight easier and your body feels much younger.

Fifty is also the age when you need to stay in shape but find it more difficult to do so. At this age, one of the best things you can do for yourself is to eat healthily. Your body will appreciate every healthy meal you give it and you are sure to enjoy the benefits extensively.

Unfortunately, eating healthily is one of the hardest things to do. There are tons of diets out there but few of them are actually practical. The Keto diet is one of those few. In this book, I'll take you on a journey of discovery through everything you need to know about Keto after 50 plus 101 awesome recipes that I live by. Eating healthily has never been easier!

# Chapter 1: What is Keto Diet?

The keto diet is one of the most popular weight loss trends sweeping the nation. The reason for its increasing popularity is due to the key benefits such as weight loss, fights against chronic diseases, increased energy and appetite control. Sounds good? In this first chapter, you will learn the essentials of the ketogenic diet which includes:

What Exactly is the Ketogenic Diet?

Everything You Need to Know About Ketosis and Ketones

Signs and Symptoms to Know You Are in Ketosis

Best Tips to Successfully Follow the Keto Diets

Thinking about starting the keto diet? Take the first step by keeping reading!

## What Exactly is the Ketogenic Diet?

What's all the fuss about the ketogenic diet? The ketogenic diet is a low carb diet that thrives on the consumption of healthy fats while decreasing your carb intake. Your daily consumption of energy comes from 75% of healthy fats, 20% from protein, and only 5% from carbohydrates. This basically means you will consume 20 to 50 grams of carbohydrates per day.

Instead of starving yourself, you are merely depriving the body of carbs. This can result in rapid weight loss, improved mental clarity, improved focus and overall better physical health. The moment you switch fuel sources, your body's metabolism changes, making you feel more energized!

The ketogenic diet is very like the Atkins diet and other low-carb ways of eating. When you switch up the sources of fuel, your body's metabolism also changes, making you feel more energized!

## Know About Ketosis and Ketones

As we mentioned before, ketosis is the metabolic state where your body uses fat as the primary source of fuel instead of sugar. The body can only transform into the state of ketosis if glycogen stored in your muscles are used up and blood sugar is low. The best way to achieve this is to follow a low-carb diet or fast until you experience symptoms of ketosis. Ketosis is hailed as an effective quick way to burn body fat and studies indicate that ketosis can positively impact our health in various ways.

How does ketosis work? Usually, your body is energized using sugar acquired from carbohydrates. However, if you extremely limit your carb intake, your body will force itself into reserved glucose, known as glycogen. Once glycogen is depleted, which typically takes 3 days, your liver will enter the process known as ketogenesis to utilize fat and produce ketone bodies. Ketone bodies are byproducts of burning fat in the body.

## Signs and Symptoms to Know You Are in Ketosis

There are several signs and symptoms to detect whether you are in the state of ketosis. Check out these symptoms to figure out if you've achieved ketosis:

If you are feeling thirstier or having a dry mouth.

If you are feeling less hungry.

If you are experiencing quick weight loss.

If you have smelly breath.

If you find yourself with reduced brain fog and increased focus.

If you are experiencing the keto flu or increased fatigue.

If you are experiencing digestive problems.

If you are experiencing insomnia.

There are three methods to check if you are in ketosis:

Measure the level of ketones in your blood by a *blood ketone meters*.

Measure the level of ketones in your urine using *urine strips*.

Measure the level of ketones in your breath using *breath ketone meters*.

# Best Tips to Successfully Follow the Keto Diet

The main goal of the ketogenic diet is to maintain the metabolic state of ketosis. This can be rather difficult for some. Below you will learn some useful tips and tricks that will help you stick to the keto diet as best as you can.

***Counting Carbs***: Keep track of your carb intake. If your consumption of carbs exceeds your daily limit, you will find it difficult to reach the state of ketosis.

Thoroughly read the nutrition information and food ingredients before purchasing ***a food product to avoid hidden sugars.***

***Clean your kitchen***: To avoid the temptation of eating sugary or high carb food you should restock your kitchen and donate bread, pasta, grains, rice, chocolate, sugary drink, etc. and replace them with low-carb alternatives.

***Have prepared keto-compliant meals at the go***. Sometimes you will unexpectedly feel hungry, which means you should have keto-friendly snacks such as kale chips, string cheese, nuts, seeds, peanut butter, celery sticks or other vegetables at the go.

***Practice intermittent fasting***. Intermittent fasting is a dieting pattern that involves fasting and then eating for a destined period of time. When you fast, your body no longer has any available fuel to use for energy, which means it must metabolize energy from the fat reserved in your body. This will result in quicker weight loss.

**Remain well hydrated.** Drinking plenty of water can help speed up your metabolism and make you feel better overall. It also helps to eliminate cravings, lessen hunger, decreases kidney stress and helps with keto breath.

**Don't overdo it with the protein.** It's a common mistake for dieters to consume too much protein. If you eat too much protein on the keto diet, you will find it harder to maintain the state of ketosis. This is due to your body converting additional protein it doesn't need into glycogen, which prevents the body from successfully entering ketosis.

Salt is crucial for specific bodily functions which include adequate digestion, potassium absorption, and maintains body fluids. On the ketogenic diet, **you should aim to consume 2 teaspoons of salt per day**. The best sources are salted cheese or butter but can also come from regular table salt as well.

**Get your carbs from quality sources.** On average, keto dieters will need to keep their consumption of net carbs under 20 to 35 grams per day. You can find good kinds of carbohydrates from starchy vegetables and fruits rather than cereal, rice, corn, wheat, etc.

# Chapter 2: Benefits of following Keto diet for Women over 50

The Keto diet has been proven to have many Benefits for people over 50. Here are some of the best.

Strengthens bones

When people get older, their bones weaken. At 50, your bones are likely not as strong as they used to be. However, you can keep them in really good condition. Consuming milk to get calcium cannot do enough to strengthen your bones. What you can do, is to make use of the Keto diet as it is low in toxins. Toxins negatively affect the absorption of nutrients and so with this, your bones can take in all they need.

Eradicates inflammation

Few things are worse than the pain from an inflamed joint or muscle. Arthritis, for instance, can be extremely difficult to bear. When you follow the ketosis diet, the production of cytokines will be reduced. Cytokines cause inflammation and therefore, their eradication will reduce it.

It eradicates nutrients deficiency

Keto focuses on consuming exactly what you need. If you use a great Keto plan, your body will lack no nutrients and will not suffer any deficiency.

Reduced hunger

The reason we find it difficult to stick to diets is hunger. It doesn't matter your age; diets do not become easier. We may have a mental picture of the healthy body we want. We may even have clear visuals of the kind of life we want to lead once free from unhealthy living but none of that matters when hunger enters the scene. However, the Keto diet is a diet that combats this problem. The Keto diet focuses on consuming plenty of proteins. Proteins are filling and do not let you feel hungry too easily. In addition, when your carb levels are reduced, your appetite takes a hit. It is a win-win situation.

Weight loss

Keto not only burns fat, but it also reduces that craving for food. Combined, these are two great ways to lose weight. It is one of the diets that has proven to help the most when it comes to weight loss. The Keto diet has been proven to be one of the best ways to burn stubborn belly fat while keeping yourself revitalized and healthy.

Reduces blood sugar and insulin

After 50, monitoring blood sugar can be a real struggle. Cutting down on carbs drastically reduces both insulin levels and blood sugar levels. This means that the Keto diet will benefit millions as a lot of people struggle with insulin complications and high blood sugar levels. It has been proven to help as when some people embark on Keto, they cut up to half of the carbs they consume. It's a treasure for those with diabetes and insulin resistance. A study was carried out on people with type 2 diabetes. After cutting down on carbs, within six months, 95 percent of people were able to reduce or totally stop using their glucose-lowering medication.

Lower levels of triglycerides

A lot of people do not know what triglycerides are. Triglycerides are molecules of fat in your blood. They are known to circulate the bloodstream and can be very dangerous. High levels of triglycerides can cause heart failures and heart diseases. However, Keto is known to reduce these levels.

Reduces acne

Although acne is mostly suffered by those who are young, there are cases of people above 50 having it. Moreover, Keto is not only for persons after 50. Acne is not only caused by blocked pores. There are quite a number of things proven to cause it. One of these things is your blood sugar. When you consume processed and refined carbs, it affects gut bacteria and results in the fluctuation of blood sugar levels. When the gut bacteria and sugar levels are affected, the skin suffers. However, when you embark on the Keto diet, you cut off on carbs intake which means that in the very first place, your gut bacteria will not be affected thereby cutting off that avenue to develop.

Increases hdl levels

HDL refers to high-density lipoprotein. When your HDL levels are compared to your LDL levels and are not found low, your risk of developing a heart disease is lowered. This is great for persons over 50 as heart diseases suddenly become more probable. Eating fats and reducing your intake of carbohydrates is one of the most assured ways to increase your high-density lipoprotein levels.

Reduces ldl levels

High levels of LDL can be very problematic when you attain 50. This is because LDL refers to bad cholesterol. People with high levels of this cholesterol are more likely to get heart attacks. When you reduce the number of carbs you consume, you will increase the size of bad LDL particles. However, this will result in the reduction of the total LDL particles as they would have increased in size. Smaller LDL particles have been linked to heart diseases while larger ones have been proven to have lower risks attached.

May help combat cancer

I termed this under 'may' because research on this is not as extensive and conclusive as we would like it to be. However, there is proof supporting it. Firstly, it helps reduce the levels of blood sugar which in turn reduces insulin complications which in turn reduces the risk of developing cancers related to insulin levels. In addition, Keto places more oxidative stress on cancer cells than on normal cells thereby making it great for chemotherapy. The risk of developing cancer after fifty is still existent and so, Keto is literally a lifesaver.

May lower blood pressure

High blood pressure plagues adults much more than it does young ones. Once you attain 50, you must monitor your blood pressure rates. Reduction in the intake of carbohydrates is a proven way to lower your blood pressure. When you cut down on your carbs and lower your blood sugar levels, you greatly reduce your chances of getting some other diseases.

Combats metabolic syndrome

As you grow older, you may find that you struggle to control your blood sugar level. Metabolic syndrome is another condition that has been proven to have an influence on diabetes and heart disease development. The symptoms associated with metabolic syndrome include but are not limited to high triglycerides, obesity, high blood sugar level, and low levels of high-density lipoprotein cholesterol.

However, you will find that reducing your level of carbohydrate intake greatly affects this. You will improve your health and majorly attack all the above-listed symptoms. Keto diet helps to fight against metabolic syndrome which is a big win.

Great for the heart

People over the age of 50 have been proven to have more chances of developing heart diseases. Keto diet has been proven to be great for the heart. As it increases good cholesterol levels and reduces the levels of bad cholesterol, you will find that partaking in the Keto diet proves extremely beneficial for your health.

May reduce seizure risks

When you change your intake levels the combination of protein, fat, and carbs, as we explained before, your body will go into ketosis. Ketosis has been proven to reduce seizure levels in people who suffer from epilepsy. When they do not respond to treatment, the ketosis treatment is used. This has been done for decades.

Combats brain disorders

Keto doesn't end there, it also combats Alzheimer's and Parkinson's disease. There are some parts of your brain that can only burn glucose and so, your body needs it. If you do not consume carbs, your lover will make use of protein to produce glucose. Your brain can also burn ketones. Ketones are formed when your carb level is very low. With this, the ketogenic diet has been used f r plenty of years to treat epilepsy in children who aren't responding to drugs. For adults, it can work the same magic as it is now being linked to treating Alzheimer's and Parkinson's disease

## Helps women suffering from polycystic ovarian syndrome (pcos)

This syndrome affects women of all ages. PCOS is short for polycystic ovarian syndrome. Polycystic ovarian syndrome is an endocrine disorder that results in enlarged ovaries with cysts. These cysts are dangerous and cause other complications. It has been proven that a high intake of carbohydrates negatively affects women suffering from polycystic ovarian syndrome. When a woman with PCOS cuts down on carbs and embarks on the Keto diet, the polycystic ovarian syndrome falls under attack.

It is beyond doubt that the Keto diet is beneficial in so many ways that it almost looks unreal. If you are to embark on the Keto diet, there are several things you must know.

# Chapter 3: Guidelines and rules for eating in the Keto Diet

A typical breakdown of a keto diet would be Fat: 70%, Carbs: 5%, and Protein: 25%.

Your daily net carbs intake should be 20-30 gram to stay in Ketosis.

Limit your fruit consumption to avocados, berries, and coconut.

Drink more water. You need to drink 2-3 litres of water daily.

Say no to carb dressings, spreads, sweeteners, or high carb nuts.

Make sure you are eating no carbs at all, and also keep track of your meal intake.

Eat fatty breakfast and eat one fat in each meal.

Stock your pantry with healthy foods, i.e., meat, eggs, starchy vegetables, avocados, saturated fats, like, coconut oil, ghee, olive oil, sesame oil, flaxseed oil.

Eat raw dairy, but if you are allergic, avoid it.

Soak and dehydrate nuts before you eat them.

Drink Bone Broth every day.

Increase your electrolytes (sodium, magnesium, and potassium) intake to keep yourself safe from Keto flu.

Plan and track your diet carefully.

# Chapter 4: What to Eat and What to Avoid

## What to Eat

1. Fats and Oils

Fats play a big role when it comes to weight loss with one of these roles being making foods that you consume better for you. How is that? Well, for starters, some nutrients and vitamins like vitamins A, D, E, and K are fat-soluble. This essentially means that you need some fat for your body to use them efficiently. In other words, if you don't take fats, your body won't be able to utilize them since they will be unavailable for the cells (the fat helps in facilitating the absorption of these vitamins). As you are already aware, in case the body cannot absorb nutrients as required, you develop nutrient deficiencies, which could come with such complications like blood clots, muscle pains, brittle bones and blindness among others.

More precisely, the vitamins mentioned above are useful in sustaining energy production, muscle health and focus; all which facilitate weight loss. For instance, vitamin E is an antioxidant while vitamin D may help the body utilize fat that occurs at the abdominal region.

In the Ketogenic diet, fat works as alternative source of energy and indeed helps trigger ketosis process or breakdown of fats into energy. To facilitate weight loss, you should take fats and oils rich in omega 3 fatty oils, from sources like salmon, tuna and trout. You are required to include both saturated and mono-saturated fats like avocados, egg yolks, butter, macadamia nuts and coconut oils as these are healthier. Unlike Tran's fats found in hardened oils, these fats have a stable chemical structure, which is less inflammatory. Thus for regular cooking such as frying your food, go for non-hydrogenated options like ghee and coconut oil.

You should also replace your regular cooking oil with coconut oil because it is rich in fatty acids known as **medium chain fatty acids**. These fatty acids have a greater satiating effect and can make you eat less and burn the stubborn fat especially in the abdomen. Examples of fat and oils that you should reach for include:

Chicken fat

Butter

Peanut butter

Avocado

Coconut oil

Non hydrogenated lard

Olive oil

2. Proteins

Protein forms a significant part of the Keto diet plan, as it helps in the synthesis and monitoring of hormones in the bloodstream. Hormones control bodily functions.

In Keto diet, good sources of protein include eggs, fish and meat. While any meat is protein-rich, a few rules should be followed when choosing your source of meat. The rule of the thumb is to go for organic and grass feed meat in place of that grain-fed meat, as corn fed to domestic animals is genetically modified, rich in hormones and antibiotics. For this reason, go for all-natural beef, pork or mutton as well as organic and free-range turkey or chicken.

When it comes to bacon, go for nitrate-free bacon and that without other additives; and wild-caught fish as opposed to the farm reared.

Here is a complete list of protein foods:

Lean Meats

Beef

Chicken

Turkey

Pork

Lamb

Game meat

Pork

Bacon

Seafood and Fish

Haddock

Trout

Shrimp

Salmon

Catfish

Tuna

Mackerel

Codfish

Poultry

Turkey: whole, breast, leg portions, or ground

Quail

Pre-cooked Rotisserie Chicken

Pre-cooked chicken strips

Pheasant

Goose

Duck

Deli meats: Turkey, Chicken, no nitrates

Cornish Hens

Chicken, whole and whole cut-up

Chicken Tenders

Canned Chicken

Chicken pieces: breasts, wings, thighs, legs

***Pork***

Sausages

Pork Tenderloin

Pork Steaks

Pork Roasts

Pork Chops

Italian Sausage

Ham

Ground Pork

Deli – Ham

Bacon

## 3. Veggies

Veggies such as kales, broccoli, and spinach are sources of vitamins and minerals; and they are low-carb and satiating. Try the following veggies and other dark leafy greens such as those listed here:

Onions

Tomatoes

Garlic

Asparagus

Collard greens

Broccoli

Parsley

Peppers

Carrots

Cauliflower

Cabbage

Spinach

Turnips

Kales

## 4. Low carb Fruits

While fruits are very nutritious and satiating, it is advisable to eat them in moderation particularly if trying to lose weight. This is because fruits contain fructose, a type of sugar that could easily get you out of ketosis and make you gain weight. Therefore, don't over-indulge in fruits; rather, limit your intake to around 1-2 fruit servings daily.

Likewise, avoid starchy fruits and fruit juices, as these have very high concentrations of carbs and sugars. When eaten in moderation, the following fruits are healthy and nutritious:

Oranges

Apples

Avocadoes

Pears

Berries (all types)

Pineapples

Papaya

## 5. Nuts and Seeds

For nuts and seeds, these are rich in healthy and satiating omega-3 fatty acids but should be moderated too as they tend to be high in carbs. Try eating these foods as snacks occasionally:

Walnuts

Macadamia nuts

Hazelnuts

Pumpkin seeds

Sunflower seeds

Flax seed

Almonds

6. Dairy

While it may come as great surprise, you should not drink or use milk in its natural form. This is because cow's milk contains allergens such as lactose (a form of sugar) that some dieters are intolerant to. But for cheese, yoghurt and other fermented dairy products, these are Ketogenic friendly and should form a large part of your diet. However, if you cannot keep off milk, try almond or coconut milk as these are suitable for blending other ingredients and actually improve the milk flavor. Try the following dairy alternatives:

Cheese

Butter

Ricotta cheese

Full Fat Cheese, use sparingly

Almond Milk

Greek or plain yogurt

Full Fat Cottage Cheese

Butter

Cream, or whipped cream

Coconut Milk

7. Spices

You should be very careful about the spices you use, as some have high concentrations of carbohydrates. Even the common table salt is usually mixed with powdered dextrose; you might want to consider using sea salt. Here is a list of spices that are good for low carb diets.

Sea salt

Black pepper

Cinnamon

Chili powder

Turmeric

Parsley

Rosemary

Sage

8. Beverages

One of the effects of being on a ketogenic diet is that you will get very dehydrated. Therefore, it is extremely important that you take plenty of water. You should also drink other liquids like coffee and tea. However, you must be careful not to drink any liquids that contain sugar, as these will jeopardize your chances of getting into ketosis and staying there. That's why it is best to avoid sugary beverages altogether. However, if you crave for something sweet, use artificial sweeteners. Try to go after liquid artificial sweeteners, as they do not have binders such as dextrose that contain carbs. Examples of sweeteners include:

Stevia

Suclarose

Erythritol

Xylitol

Monk fruit

With a wide variety of foods to enjoy, you should avoid those foods rich in processed fats, high in carb or those synthetically made and opt for organic ingredients. Here are foods that you should keep out of your pantry:

## What To Avoid

1. All grains

These include rice, wheat, barley and oats; along with products that come from them such as crackers, bagels, cereal, pasta, granola bars and bread. Simply avoid every food material that has grain in it, whether whole-grain, processed grains or whatever kind of grains you can come across. Instead, try almond or coconut flour, as these have low carb content, has high fiber level and are rich in proteins.

2. Starchy veggies

Leafy dark leafy greens are Keto friendly but avoid their starchy variety. These include popcorn, tortillas, corn chips, potatoes chips, corn and white potatoes.

3. Beans or legumes

The ketogenic diet limits intake of carbs to at most 50 grams daily so you must avoid all high carb foods such as beans and legumes for that matter. To further control your carb intake, you shouldn't eat spaghetti squash, pumpkins, acorn, butternut squash, summer squash and sweet potatoes.

## 4. Sugary foods and drinks

High carb foods and drinks include candies, cookies, sport drinks, cakes, honey, soda, syrup and jam or jelly. These may spike blood sugar, disrupt insulin function and can trigger unnecessary cravings a few hours after eating. Also avoid fruit juices at all costs, as they tend to have too much sugar and thus cannot be Keto friendly.

## 5. Vegetable oils

Although the Ketogenic diet is high in fat, this doesn't mean you can eat all fats. Avoid vegetable oils such as sunflower oil, corn oil, safflower and other hydrogenated oils. These are comprised of Tran's fats, which are linked to cardiovascular problems.

## 6. High carb drinks

Here are a number of drinks that you should stay away from:

Beers

Beers are a product of grain, which has high carb content. Alcohol also slows fat burning. If you have to drink, take low carb beers like vodka, tequila, whiskey, gin, rum, cognac and brandy.

Non diet sodas

Sweetened soda pops contain large amounts of fructose; a type of carbohydrate found in most fruits. For example, corn syrup has lots of carbs that you should avoid.

Fruit Juices

These juices concentrate sugar of the original fruit, which means you get even higher carb levels than with fresh fruits.

That said, it doesn't really mean that you forget your preferred foods among them the wheat flour, pasta, rice or other delicious starchy veggies like sweet potatoes. In fact, you can still enjoy alternative or substitutes for these foods with the same delicious and satiating effect. Here is a list of food substitutes that can help you stick to Keto diet:

# Chapter 5: Advice away from Home

Stress is a side effect of living. We get so stressed with work, school, family, our lives, etc. that we are left pulling our hair out by the time mealtime rolls around. We live for that 30-minute lunch break when we know that we can get our mind off of work. The increasing blood glucose concentrations signal the body to secrete insulin from the beta cells of the pancreas. The role of insulin in this case is to help the cells to take up glucose as the glucose-rich blood flows in different parts of the body. It (insulin) does that by triggering the insulin receptors on different cells, which in turn signals the cells to sort of 'open up' in order to take up glucose, which is then used for energy.

How many times have you looked into your fridge and sighed, knowing that there was no nutritious food for you to eat? You rummage through the ingredients you have on hand and realize that you can eat another plain apple or you have to make a full meal. No one has time to cook a full meal every time you are hungry! So then comes along a third option, go out to eat fast food. You are irked that you've already had fast food multiple times this week but the thought of cooking a full meal is stressful as well! You can't seem to catch a break.

Situations like these are what attracts most people to meal prepping. As mentioned before, meal prepping is a huge stress relief. Say goodbye to worrying about each meal! Relieving stress is probably the number one reason that people start looking into meal prepping. Why stress out about every meal and snack with junk food when you can prepare it ahead of time so that there's always food waiting for you in the refrigerator?

But how does meal prepping really reduce your stress? It's understandable that prepping all your food ahead of time could be an added stressor in your life. What will you eat? How will you cook it all? Will it even taste good? That's what these next chapters in this book are for. Starting a new food prepping routine can be overwhelming and stressful. This book aims to relieve that stress and help you meal prep in the easiest way. You won't feel an ounce of stress if you follow our guidelines and recipes!

There are many ways that meal prepping can help your stress levels. Firstly, meal prepping forces you to have a plan. There is fun in spontaneity, but we can all admit that when you have a plan, there is less stress. Humans like to know how things are going to happen and when things are going to happen. Therefore, we thrive when we create plans. When you meal prep, you create a plan for the next week or month. You don't have to worry about what you are going to make for your meals, and you don't have to spend time each day figuring out the plan for your meals. You will not have to stress when lunchtime or dinnertime comes around because your meal will already be cooked. This is a huge stress relief not only for the single individuals, but also especially for those with a family.

Providing food for a family can be one of the most stressful things you do! You don't want to cook them unhealthy options and you most definitely don't want to cook the same thing every week.

Having a plan isn't the only benefit to meal prepping. When you plan your meals, you also plan your groceries. Going to the grocery store can be overwhelming. How many times have you gone to the store, picked up your groceries, and then arrived home realizing you forget a few items? Too many times! You try to write a list for the upcoming week but if you don't know what meals you are planning to make, how can you make a correct grocery list? You can't. So when you arrive home, you realize you forgot a few items, and now you are immediately stressed that you have to go back to the store. With meal prepping, this doesn't happen. You go to the store with a grocery list in hand and you leave the store with only the items you need. This leads to a lot lesser stress.

"You're late! You're late! For a very important date!" You check your clock and realize that time has passed you by. You spent a little too long getting ready and now you either have to go hungry or grab something on the way to work because you don't have time to make a meal. You decide that you are going to hit up the drive through once you hear your stomach grumbling. You get to the drive through line, and guess what? The line is long! Is it worth getting the food? You tap your foot and keep glancing at the clock, fully aware that time is ticking away. Your stomach is grumbling, you're going to be late for your first meeting, and you still haven't ordered your food. By the time you do finally get your food, it is mediocre and doesn't taste nearly as good as you thought it would. It's going to be a long day.

Would you believe that prepping your food in advance will actually save you time each day? While it may take a little bit of time upfront to prepare and get the food ready for the week, you'll save time in the long run. Let's rewind that situation.

You check the clock and realize time has passed you by. Once again, you spent too long getting ready for the day. You hurry and finish getting ready. Before you leave, you open your refrigerator. Shining in the light is your delicious meal prepped breakfast. You smile to yourself as your grab what you need, and head out the door. As you drive to work you see the long drive through line. You smile to yourself knowing that you don't have to wait in that line. You walk through your office doors with five minutes to spare before your first meeting. Score.

Meal prepping can save you a ton of time. It's easy to prepare beforehand and when the time matters, you won't have to waste it waiting in a drive through or cooking up a huge meal. You can sit down, eat and then go!

When you create a plan and meal prep, you will spend less time cooking dinner, which leaves you more time for your family. You can sit down once a week and make your meal plan for the week. Or, you can sit down once a month and create a meal plan for the whole month. How you do it is up to you. Sure, you'll spend maybe an hour getting your plan ready for the month, but you'll save that time every single day when you try and craft up a meal for dinner. You won't have to think and worry about what to cook. And then cooking is also easier. If you choose to do the freezer prep route, you'll spend 5 minutes in the morning putting your meal into your slow cooker. When you get home from work or wrangling in the kids from school, your meal will be ready to eat! No more slaving over a hot stove and oven. It's truly a win-win situation.

# Chapter 6: Measurement conversion Tables

But if you must move from stressing about work to stressing about what you'll eat for lunch, then those precious minutes of break time kiss us goodbye! And that's not where the stress ends. Upon breakdown of carbohydrates into glucose, the glucose is then absorbed into the bloodstream for transportation to different parts of the body.

The increasing blood glucose concentrations signal the body to secrete insulin from the beta cells of the pancreas. The role of insulin in this case is to help the cells to take up glucose as the glucose-rich blood flows in different parts of the body.

We have gone to great length in order to make sure that the measurements are on the following Measurement Charts are accurate.

## American and British Variances

| Term | Abbreviation | Nationality | Dry or liquid | Metric equivalent | Equivalent in context |
|------|--------------|-------------|---------------|-------------------|-----------------------|
| cup | c., C. | | usually liquid | 237 milliliters | 16 tablespoons or 8 ounces |
| ounce | fl oz, fl. oz. | American | liquid only | 29.57 milliliters | |
| | | British | either | 28.41 milliliters | |
| gallon | gal. | American | liquid only | 3.785 liters | 4 quarts |
| | | British | either | 4.546 liters | 4 quarts |
| inch | in, in. | | | 2.54 centimeters | |
| ounce | oz, oz. | American | dry | 28.35 grams | 1/16 pound |
| | | | liquid | see OUNCE | see OUNCE |
| pint | p., pt. | American | liquid | 0.473 liter | 1/8 gallon or 16 ounces |
| | | | dry | 0.551 liter | 1/2 quart |
| | | British | either | 0.568 liter | |
| pound | lb. | | dry | 453.592 grams | 16 ounces |
| Quart | q., qt, qt. | American | liquid | 0.946 liter | 1/4 gallon or 32 ounces |
| | | | dry | 1.101 liters | 2 pints |
| | | British | either | 1.136 liters | |
| Teaspoon | t., tsp., tsp | | either | about 5 milliliters | 1/3 tablespoon |
| Tablespoon | T., tbs., tbsp. | | either | about 15 milliliters | 3 teaspoons or 1/2 ounce |

## Volume (Liquid)

| American Standard (Cups & Quarts ) | American Standard (Ounces) | Metric (Milliliters & Liters) |
|-----------------------------------|----------------------------|-------------------------------|
| 2 tbsp. | 1 fl. oz. | 30 ml |
| 1/4 cup | 2 fl. oz. | 60 ml |
| 1/2 cup | 4 fl. oz. | 125 ml |
| 1 cup | 8 fl. oz. | 250 ml |
| 1 1/2 cups | 12 fl. oz. | 375 ml |
| 2 cups or 1 pint | 16 fl. oz. | 500 ml |
| 4 cups or 1 quart | 32 fl. oz. | 1000 ml or 1 liter |
| 1 gallon | 128 fl. oz. | 4 liters |

## Volume (Dry)

| American Standard | Metric |
|---|---|
| 1/8 teaspoon | 5 ml |
| 1/4 teaspoon | 1 ml |
| 1/2 teaspoon | 2 ml |
| 3/4 teaspoon | 4 ml |
| 1 teaspoon | 5 ml |
| 1 tablespoon | 15 ml |
| 1/4 cup | 59 ml |
| 1/3 cup | 79 ml |
| 1/2 cup | 118 ml |
| 2/3 cup | 158 ml |
| 3/4 cup | 177 ml |
| 1 cup | 225 ml |
| 2 cups or 1 pint | 450 ml |
| 3 cups | 675 ml |
| 4 cups or 1 quart | 1 liter |
| 1/2 gallon | 2 liters |
| 1 gallon | 4 liters |

## Oven Temperatures

| American Standard | Metric |
|---|---|
| 250° F | 130° C |
| 300° F | 150° C |
| 350° F | 180° C |
| 400° F | 200° C |
| 450° F | 230° C |

## Weight (Mass)

| American Standard (Ounces) | Metric (Grams) |
|---|---|
| 1/2 ounce | 15 grams |
| 1 ounce | 30 grams |
| 3 ounces | 85 grams |
| 3.75 ounces | 100 grams |
| 4 ounces | 115 grams |
| 8 ounces | 225 grams |
| 12 ounces | 340 grams |
| 16 ounces or 1 pound | 450 grams |

## Dry Measure Equivalents

| | | | |
|---|---|---|---|
| 3 teaspoons | 1 tablespoon | 1/2 ounce | 14.3 grams |
| 2 tablespoons | 1/8 cup | 1 ounce | 28.3 grams |
| 4 tablespoons | 1/4 cup | 2 ounces | 56.7 grams |
| 5 1/3 tablespoons | 1/3 cup | 2.6 ounces | 75.6 grams |
| 8 tablespoons | 1/2 cup | 4 ounces | 113.4 grams |
| 12 tablespoons | 3/4 cup | 6 ounces | .375 pound |
| 32 tablespoons | 2 cups | 16 ounces | 1 pound |

# Chapter 7: Nutritional Value of all meals

Macro is the short form of macronutrients (fats, proteins and carbohydrates). These macros are the basis of calories that you consume.

Calculating your macronutrients and total calories is very important on Ketogenic diet. First calculating macros will look really tough, but it is actually really easy once you understand it.

Everyone is different so macros are different for everyone. Total calories are different for everyone. Those who live really active lifestyle will need more calories than those who don't work out at all.

When calculating macros, the first step is to calculate your TDEE (Total Daily Energy Expenditure). It is basically total number of calories that you burn in a day. If you eat less than your total daily energy expenditure then you will lose weight, but if you eat more than your total daily energy expenditure then you will gain weight.

BASIC FORMULA

In this formula first we will calculate your energy expenditure when you are resting, that is energy required to run your body when you don't move at all.

Since most people do move and not just lie in their bed, next we have to find expenditure of their movements.

**Sedentary**

Walking, talking, eating etc. Normal day to day mundane activities. (REE x 1.1)

Light activity

Activities which burn around 200-400 calories for women and 250-500 calories for men come under light activity. (REE x 1.38)

Moderate activity

Activities which burns 400-650 calories for women and 500-800 calories for men comes under moderate activity. (REE x 1.6).

Very active

Activities which burn more than 651 calories for women and more than 801 calories for men comes under very active.( REE x 1.8).

A typical TDEE equation is like this

Let's say you are 30 years old, 184 cm, 90 kgs, very active man

These will be your results

(10 x weight (kg) + 6.24 x height (cm) − 5 x age (y) + 6 = REE) x 1.8 = TDEE

10 x 90 + 6.24 x 184 − 5 x 30 + 6 = REE

900 + 1148.16 − 150 + 6 = REE

1904.16 = REE

1904.16 x 1.8 = 3427.488

TDEE = 3427.488

If your Total daily energy expenditure is 3427.488.

If you will eat more than this, you will gain weight.

If you eat exactly 3427 calories than you will neither lose weight nor will you gain weight.

If you will eat less than 3427 calories then you will lose weight for sure.

Losing weight

If you want to lose weight then I will recommend don't drop your calories more than 20 % of your total daily energy expenditure. This way you will have enough energy to carry out your mundane tasks and live life with ease. You will stick to your diet but if you drop your calories too much than you will become demotivated and irritated by this diet and you will find yourself binge eating.

Gaining weight

Same goes with gaining weight, increase your calories by 20 %. This way you will gain lean muscles and will stay in control of your life.

## MACROS

First step was getting your TDEE. Now we will calculate macronutrients that make up your diet.

1gram of protein = 4 calories.

1 gram of fat = 9 calories.

1 gram of carbohydrates = 4 calories.

So suppose you want to lose weight and your TDEE is 2000 calories per day.

You will consume around 1600 calories (2000 – 20 % of 2000).

## FATS

Now 70 % of 1600 will be from fats.

70 % of 1600 = 1120.

1120 / 9 = 124 grams (1 gram of fats = 9 calories)

1120 Calories of fats means 124 grams of fats.

## PROTEINS

25 % will be from proteins.

So 25 % of 1600 = 400 calories.

400/4 = 100 grams of proteins will be consumed.

## CARBOHYDRATES

5% OF 1600 calories will be from carbohydrates which will be around 80 grams of carbohydrates. But try to lower your carbohydrate intake overtime; it should get below 50 grams per day.

# Chapter 8: Shopping List

Following are the foods that are emphasized on a keto diet.

Healthy, fatty fish such as tuna, salmon, etc.

Healthy oils such as avocado oil, coconut oil, olive oil, etc.

All types of full-fat cheese and full-fat cream cheese, sour cream, crème Fraiche.

Unsweetened almond/coconut milk, or other nut milk

Eggs

Butter, total fat

Avocados

Walnuts, almonds, cashews, and other nuts

Chia seed and flax seed

Olives

Bacon

Unsweetened beverages

Heavy cream

Healthy low carb, non-starchy veggies such as leek, fennel, spinach, kale, broccoli, tomatoes, other greens, etc.

All types of berries but in small quantities

Herbs and most spices

# Chapter 9: 30 Day Meal Plan

## Day 1

Starters Recipes - Minty Green Chicken Salad

First Course Recipes - Tangy Steamed Artichokes

Second Course Recipes - Enticing Chicken and Broccoli Casserole

## Day 2

Starters Recipes - Spinach Salad with Goat Cheese & Pine Nuts

First Course Recipes - Succulent Sausage and Cheese Dip

Second Course Recipes - Italian-Inspired Chicken Breast

## Day 3

Starters Recipes - Salmon Salad with Lettuce & Avocado

First Course Recipes - Ravishing Mushrooms and Sausage Gravy

Second Course Recipes - Energetic Lemon Chicken

## Day 4

Starters Recipes - Classic Greek Salad

First Course Recipes - Flawless Cranberry Sauce

Second Course Recipes - Excellent Creamy Chicken

## Day 5

Starters Recipes - Kale & Broccoli Slaw Salad with Bacon & Parmesan

First Course Recipes - Very Cheesy Cheese Sauce

Second Course Recipes - Definite Pecan-Crusted Chicken

## Day 6

Starters Recipes - Seared Rump Steak Salad

First Course Recipes - Best Homemade Alfredo Sauce

Second Course Recipes - Flavorsome Pulled Pork

## Day 7

Starters Recipes - Spinach Salad with Bacon & Mustard Vinaigrette

First Course Recipes - Knockout Asparagus and Shrimp Mix

Second Course Recipes - Hearty Lemon & Garlic Pork

## Day 8

Starters Recipes - Minty Green Chicken Salad

First Course Recipes - Tangy Steamed Artichokes

Second Course Recipes - Enticing Chicken and Broccoli Casserole

## Day 9

Starters Recipes - Spinach Salad with Goat Cheese & Pine Nuts

First Course Recipes - Succulent Sausage and Cheese Dip

Second Course Recipes - Italian-Inspired Chicken Breast

## Day 10

Starters Recipes - Salmon Salad with Lettuce & Avocado

First Course Recipes - Ravishing Mushrooms and Sausage Gravy

Second Course Recipes - Energetic Lemon Chicken

## Day 11

Starters Recipes - Classic Greek Salad

First Course Recipes - Flawless Cranberry Sauce

Second Course Recipes - Excellent Creamy Chicken

## Day 12

Starters Recipes - Kale & Broccoli Slaw Salad with Bacon & Parmesan

First Course Recipes - Very Cheesy Cheese Sauce

Second Course Recipes - Definite Pecan-Crusted Chicken

## Day 13

Starters Recipes - Seared Rump Steak Salad

First Course Recipes - Best Homemade Alfredo Sauce

Second Course Recipes - Flavorsome Pulled Pork

## Day 14

Starters Recipes - Spinach Salad with Bacon & Mustard Vinaigrette

First Course Recipes - Knockout Asparagus and Shrimp Mix

Second Course Recipes - Hearty Lemon & Garlic Pork

## Day 15

Starters Recipes - Minty Green Chicken Salad

First Course Recipes - Tangy Steamed Artichokes

Second Course Recipes - Enticing Chicken and Broccoli Casserole

## Day 16

Starters Recipes - Spinach Salad with Goat Cheese & Pine Nuts

First Course Recipes - Succulent Sausage and Cheese Dip

Second Course Recipes - Italian-Inspired Chicken Breast

## Day 17

Starters Recipes - Salmon Salad with Lettuce & Avocado

First Course Recipes - Ravishing Mushrooms and Sausage Gravy

Second Course Recipes - Energetic Lemon Chicken

## Day 18

Starters Recipes - Classic Greek Salad

First Course Recipes - Flawless Cranberry Sauce

Second Course Recipes - Excellent Creamy Chicken

## Day 19

Starters Recipes - Kale & Broccoli Slaw Salad with Bacon & Parmesan

First Course Recipes - Very Cheesy Cheese Sauce

Second Course Recipes - Definite Pecan-Crusted Chicken

## Day 20

Starters Recipes - Seared Rump Steak Salad

First Course Recipes - Best Homemade Alfredo Sauce

Second Course Recipes - Flavorsome Pulled Pork

## Day 21

Starters Recipes - Spinach Salad with Bacon & Mustard Vinaigrette

First Course Recipes - Knockout Asparagus and Shrimp Mix

Second Course Recipes - Hearty Lemon & Garlic Pork

## Day 22

Starters Recipes - Minty Green Chicken Salad

First Course Recipes - Tangy Steamed Artichokes

Second Course Recipes - Enticing Chicken and Broccoli Casserole

## Day 23

Starters Recipes - Spinach Salad with Goat Cheese & Pine Nuts

First Course Recipes - Succulent Sausage and Cheese Dip

Second Course Recipes - Italian-Inspired Chicken Breast

## Day 24

Starters Recipes - Salmon Salad with Lettuce & Avocado

First Course Recipes - Ravishing Mushrooms and Sausage Gravy

Second Course Recipes - Energetic Lemon Chicken

# Day 25

Starters Recipes - Classic Greek Salad

First Course Recipes - Flawless Cranberry Sauce

Second Course Recipes - Excellent Creamy Chicken

# Day 26

Starters Recipes - Kale & Broccoli Slaw Salad with Bacon & Parmesan

First Course Recipes - Very Cheesy Cheese Sauce

Second Course Recipes - Definite Pecan-Crusted Chicken

# Day 27

Starters Recipes - Seared Rump Steak Salad

First Course Recipes - Best Homemade Alfredo Sauce

Second Course Recipes - Flavorsome Pulled Pork

# Day 28

Starters Recipes - Spinach Salad with Bacon & Mustard Vinaigrette

First Course Recipes - Knockout Asparagus and Shrimp Mix

Second Course Recipes - Hearty Lemon & Garlic Pork

# Day 29

Starters Recipes - Salmon Salad with Lettuce & Avocado

First Course Recipes - Ravishing Mushrooms and Sausage Gravy

Second Course Recipes - Energetic Lemon Chicken

# Day 30

Starters Recipes - Classic Greek Salad

First Course Recipes - Flawless Cranberry Sauce

Second Course Recipes - Excellent Creamy Chicken

# Chapter 10: Starters Recipes (20 Recipes)Feta & Sun-Dried Tomato

## Minty Green Chicken Salad

**Prep + Cook Time**: 25 minutes

**Ingredients**

1 chicken breast, cubed

1 tbsp avocado oil

2 eggs

2 cups green beans, steamed

1 avocado, sliced

4 cups mixed salad greens

2 tbsp olive oil

2 tbsp lemon juice

1 tsp Dijon mustard

1 tbsp mint, chopped

Salt and black pepper, to taste

## Directions

Boil the eggs in salted water over medium heat for 10 minutes. Remove to an ice bath to cool, peel and slice. Warm the oil in a pan over medium heat. Add the chicken and cook for about 4 minutes.

Divide the green beans between two salad bowls. Top with chicken, eggs, and avocado slices. In another bowl, whisk together the lemon juice, olive oil, mustard, salt, and pepper, and drizzle over the salad. Top with mint and serve.

# Spinach Salad with Goat Cheese & Pine Nuts

**Prep + Cook Time**: 20 minutes

## Ingredients

2 cups spinach

½ cup pine nuts

1 ½ cups hard goat cheese, grated

2 tbsp white wine vinegar

2 tbsp extra virgin olive oil

Salt and black pepper, to taste

## Directions

Preheat oven to 390 F. Place the grated goat cheese in two circles on two pieces of parchment paper. Place in the oven and bake for 10 minutes.

Find two same bowls, place them upside down, and carefully put the parchment paper on top to give the cheese a bowl-like shape. Let cool that way for 15 minutes. Divide spinach among the bowls sprinkle with salt and pepper and drizzle with vinegar and olive oil. Top with pine nuts to serve.

# Salmon Salad with Lettuce & Avocado

**Prep + Cook Time**: 5 minutes

## Ingredients

2 slices smoked salmon, chopped

1 tsp onion flakes

3 tbsp mayonnaise

1 cup romaine lettuce, shredded

1 tbsp lime juice

1 tbsp extra virgin olive oil

Sea salt to taste

½ avocado, sliced

## Directions

Combine the salmon, mayonnaise, lime juice, olive oil, and salt in a small bowl; mix to combine well.

In a salad platter, arrange the shredded lettuce and onion flakes. Spread the salmon mixture over; top with avocado slices and serve.

# Classic Greek Salad

**Prep + Cook Time**: 10 minutes

## Ingredients

3 tbsp extra virgin olive oil

½ lemon, juiced

3 tomatoes, sliced

1 cucumber, sliced

1 red bell pepper, sliced

1 small red onion, chopped

10 kalamata olives, chopped

4 oz feta cheese, cubed

1 tsp parsley, chopped

Salt to taste

## Directions

Mix the olive oil with lemon juice and salt, in a small bowl. In a salad plate, combine the tomatoes, cucumber, bell pepper and parsley; toss with the dressing. Top with the feta and olives, and serve.

# Kale & Broccoli Slaw Salad with Bacon & Parmesan

**Prep + Cook Time**: 10 minutes

## Ingredients

2 tbsp olive oil

1 cup broccoli slaw

1 cup kale slaw

2 slices bacon, chopped

2 tbsp Parmesan cheese, grated

1 tsp celery seeds

1 ½ tbsp apple cider vinegar

Salt and black pepper, to taste

## Directions

Fry the bacon in a skillet over medium heat until crispy, about 5 minutes. Set aside to cool.

Place broccoli, kale slaw and celery seeds in a large salad bowl. Pour the olive oil and vinegar over. Season with salt and black pepper, and mix with your hands to combine well. Sprinkle with the cooled bacon and Parmesan cheese, and serve.

# Seared Rump Steak Salad

**Prep + Cook Time**: 40 minutes

## Ingredients

½ cup water

½ lb rump steak

3 green onions, sliced

3 tomatoes, sliced

1 cup green beans, steamed and sliced

1 avocado, sliced

2 cups mixed salad greens

2 tsp yellow mustard

Salt and black pepper to taste

3 tbsp extra virgin olive oil

1 tbsp balsamic vinegar

## Directions

In a bowl, mix the mustard, salt, black pepper, balsamic vinegar, and extra virgin olive oil. Set aside.

Preheat a grill pan over high heat while you season the meat with salt and pepper.

Place the steak in the pan and brown on both sides for 4 minutes each. Remove to rest on a chopping board for 4 more minutes before slicing thinly.

In a shallow salad bowl, add the green onions, tomatoes, green beans, salad greens, and steak slices. Drizzle the dressing over and toss with two spoons. Top with avocado slices to serve.

# Spinach Salad with Bacon & Mustard Vinaigrette

**Prep + Cook Time**: 20 minutes

## Ingredients

1 cup spinach

1 large avocado, sliced

1 spring onion, sliced

2 bacon slices

½ lettuce head, shredded

1 hard-boiled egg, chopped

Vinaigrette:

Salt to taste

¼ tsp garlic powder

3 tbsp olive oil

1 tsp Dijon mustard

1 tbsp white wine vinegar

## Directions

Chop the bacon and fry in a skillet over medium heat for 5 minutes until crispy. Set aside to cool.

Mix the spinach, lettuce, egg, and spring onion, in a bowl. Whisk together the vinaigrette ingredients in another bowl. Pour the dressing over, toss to combine and top with avocado and bacon.

# Mackerel Lettuce Cups

**Prep + Cook Time**: 20 minutes

## Ingredients

2 mackerel fillets, cut into pieces

1 tbsp olive oil

Salt and black pepper to taste

2 eggs

1 ½ cups water

1 tomato, seeded, chopped

2 tbsp mayonnaise

½ head green lettuce, firm leaves removed for cups

## Directions

Preheat a grill pan over medium heat. Drizzle the mackerel fillets with olive oil, and sprinkle with salt and black pepper. Add the fish to the preheated grill pan and cook on both sides for 6-8 minutes.

Bring the eggs to boil in salted water in a pot over medium heat for 10 minutes. Then, run the eggs in cold water, peel, and chop into small pieces. Transfer to a salad bowl.

Remove the mackerel fillets to the salad bowl. Include the tomatoes and mayonnaise; mix evenly with a spoon. Layer two lettuce leaves each as cups and fill with two tablespoons of egg salad each.

# Classic Egg Salad with Olives

**Prep + Cook Time**: 20 minutes

## Ingredients

4 eggs

¼ cup mayonnaise

½ tsp sriracha sauce

½ tbsp mustard

¼ cup scallions

¼ stalk celery, minced

Salt and black pepper, to taste

1 head romaine lettuce, torn into pieces

¼ tsp fresh lime juice

10 black olives

## Directions

Boil the eggs in salted water over medium heat for 10 minutes. When cooled, peel and chop them into bite-size pieces. Place in a salad bowl.

Stir in the remaining ingredients, except for the scallions, until everything is well combined. Scatter the scallions all over and decorate with olives to serve.

# Spinach & Brussels Sprouts Salad with Hazelnuts

**Prep + Cook Time**: 35 minutes

## Ingredients

1 lb Brussels sprouts, halved

2 tbsp olive oil

Salt and black pepper to taste

1 tbsp balsamic vinegar

2 tbsp extra virgin olive oil

1 cup baby spinach

1 tbsp Dijon mustard

½ cup hazelnuts

## Directions

Preheat oven to 400 F. Drizzle the Brussels sprouts with olive oil, a little salt and black pepper, in a bowl, and spread on a baking sheet. Bake until tender for about 20 minutes.

In a dry pan over medium heat, toast the hazelnuts for 2-3 minutes, cool and then chop into small pieces.

Transfer the Brussels sprouts to a salad bowl and add the baby spinach, Dijon mustard and hazelnuts. Mix until well combined.

In a small bowl combine the vinegar with the olive oil. Scatter the dressing over the salad to serve.

# Mediterranean Artichoke & Red Onion Salad

**Prep + Cook Time**: 30 minutes

## Ingredients

6 baby artichoke hearts, halved

½ lemon, juiced

½ red onion, sliced

¼ cup cherry peppers, halved

¼ cup pitted olives, sliced

¼ cup olive oil

¼ tsp lemon zest

2 tsp balsamic vinegar, sugar-free

1 tbsp chopped dill

Salt and black pepper to taste

1 tbsp capers

## Directions

Bring a pot of salted water to a boil. Add the artichokes to the pot. Lower the heat, and let simmer for 20 minutes until tender. Drain and place the artichokes in a bowl.

Add in the rest of the ingredients, except for the olives; toss to combine well. Transfer to a serving platter and top with the olives.

# Tomato & Pesto Sausage Salad

**Prep + Cook Time**: 10 minutes

## Ingredients

½ pound pork sausage links, sliced

½ cup mixed cherry tomatoes, cut in half

1 cups mixed lettuce greens

¼ cup radicchio, sliced

1 tbsp olive oil

¼ pound feta cheese, cubed

½ tbsp lemon juice

½ cup basil pesto

¼ cup black olives, pitted and halved

Salt and black pepper, to taste

1 tbsp Parmesan shavings

## Directions

Cook the sausages in warm olive oil over medium heat for 4 minutes per side.

In a salad bowl, combine the mixed lettuce greens, radicchio, feta cheese, pesto, cherry tomatoes, black olives, and lemon juice, and toss well to coat.

Season with salt and black pepper and add the sausage pieces. Finish with Parmesan shavings and serve.

# Arugula Chicken Salad with Gorgonzola Cheese

**Prep + Cook Time**: 15 minutes

## Ingredients

1 chicken breast, boneless, skinless, flattened

Salt and black pepper to taste

1 tbsp garlic powder

2 tsp olive oil

1 cup arugula

1 tbsp red wine vinegar

½ cup gorgonzola cheese, crumbled

## Directions

Rub the chicken with salt, black pepper, and garlic powder. Heat half of the olive oil in a pan over high heat and fry the chicken for 4 minutes on both sides until golden brown.

Remove chicken to a cutting board and let cool before slicing.

Toss arugula with red wine vinegar and the remaining olive oil; share the salads into plates.

Divide chicken slices on top and sprinkle with gorgonzola cheese.

# Modern Greek Salad with Avocado

**Prep + Cook Time**: 10 minutes

## Ingredients

2 tomatoes, sliced

1 avocado, sliced

6 kalamata olives

¼ lb feta cheese, sliced

1 red bell pepper, roasted and sliced

1 tbsp vinegar

1 tbsp olive oil

1 tbsp parsley, chopped

## Directions

Put the tomato slices on a serving platter and place the avocado slices in the middle. Arrange the olives and bell pepper slices around the avocado slices and drop pieces of feta on the platter. Drizzle with olive oil and vinegar and sprinkle with parsley to serve.

# Pickled Pepper & Cheese Salad with Grilled Steak

**Prep + Cook Time**: 15 minutes

## Ingredients

½ cup feta cheese, crumbled

1 lb skirt steak, sliced

Salt and black pepper to season

1 tsp olive oil

1 cup watercress

1 cup arugula

3 pickled peppers, chopped

2 tbsp red wine vinegar

## Directions

Preheat grill to high heat. Season the steak slices with salt and black pepper and drizzle with olive oil. Grill the steaks on each side to the desired doneness, for about 5-6 minutes. Remove to a bowl, cover and leave to rest while you make the salad.

Mix the watercress and arugula, pickled peppers, and vinegar in a salad bowl. Add the beef and sprinkle with feta cheese.

# Watercress & Shrimp Salad with Lemon Dressing

**Prep + Cook Time**: 1 hour 10 minutes

## Ingredients

1 cup watercress leaves

2 tbsp capers

½ pound shrimp, cooked

1 tbsp dill, chopped

Dressing:

¼ cup mayonnaise

½ tsp apple cider vinegar

¼ tsp sesame seeds

Salt and black pepper to taste

1 tbsp lemon juice

2 tsp stevia

## Directions

Combine the watercress leaves, shrimp, and dill in a large bowl. Whisk together the mayonnaise, vinegar, sesame seeds, black pepper, stevia, and lemon juice in another bowl. Season with salt.

Pour the dressing over and gently toss to combine; refrigerate for 1 hour. Top with capers to serve.

# Salad of Prawns and Mixed Lettuce Greens

**Prep + Cook Time**: 15 minutes

## Ingredients

2 cups mixed lettuce greens

¼ cup aioli

1 tbsp olive oil

½ pound tiger prawns, peeled and deveined

½ tsp Dijon mustard

Salt and chili pepper to season

1 tbsp lemon juice

## Directions

Season the prawns with salt and chili pepper. Fry in warm olive oil over medium heat for 3 minutes on each side until prawns are pink. Set aside. Add the aioli, lemon juice and mustard in a small bowl. Mix until smooth and creamy.

Place the mixed lettuce greens in a bowl and pour half of the dressing on the salad. Toss with 2 spoons until mixed, and add the remaining dressing. Divide salad aming plates and serve with prawns.

# Arugula & Watercress Turkey Salad with Walnuts

**Prep + Cook Time**: 25 minutes

## Ingredients

1 tbsp xylitol

1 red onion, chopped

2 tbsp lime juice

3 tbsp olive oil

¼ cup water

1 ¾ cups raspberries

1 tbsp Dijon mustard

Salt and black pepper, to taste

1 cup arugula

1 cup watercress

1 pound turkey breasts, boneless

4 ounces goat cheese, crumbled

½ cup walnut halves

## Directions

Start with the dressing: in a blender, combine xylitol, lime juice, 1 cup raspberries, pepper, mustard, water, onion, oil, and salt, and pulse until smooth. Strain this into a bowl, and set aside.

Heat a pan over medium heat and grease lightly with cooking spray. Coat the turkey with salt and black pepper and cut in half. Place skin side down into the pan.

Cook for 8 minutes flipping to the other side and cooking for 5 minutes.

Place the arugula and watercress in a salad platter, scatter with the remaining raspberries, walnut halves, and goat cheese.

Slice the turkey breasts, put over the salad and top with raspberries dressing to serve.

# Pesto Caprese Salad with Tuna

**Prep + Cook Time**: 10 minutes

## Ingredients

1 tomato, sliced

4 oz canned tuna chunks in water, drained

1 ball fresh mozzarella cheese, sliced

4 basil leaves

½ cup pine nuts

½ cup Parmesan cheese, grated

½ cup extra virgin olive oil

½ lemon, juiced

## Directions

Put in a food processor the basil leaves, pine nuts, Parmesan cheese and extra virgin olive oil, and blend until smooth. Add in the lemon juice. Arrange the cheese and tomato slices in a serving plate. Scatter the tuna chunks and pesto over the top and serve.

# Chicken Salad with Parmesan

**Prep + Cook Time**: 30 minutes

## Ingredients

½ pound boneless, skinless chicken thighs

¼ cup lemon juice

2 garlic cloves, minced

2 tbsp olive oil

1 head romaine lettuce, shredded

3 Parmesan crisps

Parmesan cheese, grated for garnishing

Dressing:

2 tbsp extra virgin olive oil

1 tbsp lemon juice

Salt and black pepper to taste

## Directions

In a Ziploc bag, put the chicken, lemon juice, olive oil, and garlic. Seal the bag, shake to combine, and refrigerate for 1 hour.

Preheat the grill to medium heat and grill the chicken for about 4 minutes per side.

Combine the dressing ingredients in a small bowl and mix well.

On a serving platter, arrange the lettuce and Parmesan crisps. Scatter the dressing over and toss to coat. Top with the chicken and grated Parmesan cheese to serve.

# Salad with Bacon

**Prep + Cook Time**: 10 minutes

## Ingredients

3 oz bacon slices, chopped

5 sun-dried tomatoes in oil, sliced

4 basil leaves

1 cup feta cheese, crumbled

2 tsp extra virgin olive oil

1 tsp balsamic vinegar

Salt to taste

## Directions

Fry the bacon in a pan over medium heat, until golden and crisp, for about 5 minutes. Remove with a perforated spoon and set aside. Arrange the sun-dried tomatoes on a serving plate.

Scatter feta cheese over and top with basil leaves. Add the crispy bacon on top, drizzle with olive oil and sprinkle with vinegar and salt.

# Chapter 11: First Course Recipes (30 Recipes)

## Tangy Steamed Artichokes

**Prep + Cook Time**: 30 minutes

**Ingredients**

- 2 artichokes

- Juice from 1 lemon

- 2 Tablespoons low-carb mayonnaise

- 2 cups of water

- 1 teaspoon paprika

- 1 teaspoon salt (to taste)

- 1 teaspoon fresh ground black pepper (to taste)

**Directions:**

Wash and trim artichokes. Pour 2 cups of water in Instant Pot.

Place artichokes in steamer basket. Place basket in Instant Pot.

Close and seal lid. Press Manual switch. Cook at High Pressure for 10 minutes.

Release pressure naturally when done. Open the lid with care.

In a bowl, combine mayonnaise, lemon juice, paprika, salt, and black pepper. Spread on artichokes. Serve.

# Succulent Sausage and Cheese Dip

**Prep + Cook Time**: 15 minutes

## Ingredients

-       1 pound ground Italian sausage

-       ¼ cup green onions, chopped

-       1 cup cream cheese, softened

-       1 cup mozzarella cheese, shredded

-       1 cup cheddar cheese, shredded

-       1 cup vegetable broth

-       2 cups canned diced tomatoes

-       2 Tablespoons ghee, melted

## Directions:

Press Sauté button on Instant Pot. Heat the ghee.

Sauté Italian sausage and green onions, until sausage is brown.

Add remaining ingredients. Stir well.

Close and seal lid. Press Manual button. Cook at High Pressure for 5 minutes.

When the timer beeps, naturally release pressure. Open the lid with care. Serve.

# Ravishing Mushrooms and Sausage Gravy

**Prep + Cook Time**: 15 minutes

**Ingredients**

- 1 pound Italian ground sausage

- 2 Tablespoons coconut oil

- 1 yellow onion, diced

- 2 garlic cloves, minced

- 2 cups mushrooms, chopped

- 1 red bell pepper, minced

- 2 Tablespoons ghee, melted

- ⅓ cup coconut flour

- 3½ cups coconut milk, unsweetened

- ½ cup organic heavy cream

- 1 teaspoon salt (to taste)

- 1 teaspoon fresh ground black pepper (to taste)

## Directions:

Press Sauté button on Instant Pot. Heat the coconut oil. Sauté onion and garlic for 2 minutes.

Add the Italian sausage. Cook until brown.

Add mushrooms, bell peppers and sauté until soft. Season with salt and pepper.

Press Keep Warm/Cancel button to end Sauté mode.

In a small saucepan, over medium heat, melt the ghee. Add the flour. Whisk in coconut milk and heavy cream. Continue stirring until thickens. Add flour mixture to Instant Pot. Stir well.

Close and seal lid. Press Manual button. Cook at High Pressure for 10 minutes.

When the timer beeps, naturally release pressure. Open the lid with care. Serve.

# Flawless Cranberry Sauce

**Prep + Cook Time**: 20 minutes

## Ingredients

- 12-ounces fresh cranberries

- ¼ cup red wine

- 1 Tablespoon granulated Splenda

- Juice from 1 orange

- ⅛ teaspoon salt

## Directions:

Add all ingredients to Instant Pot. Stir well.

Close and seal lid. Press Manual switch. Cook at High Pressure for 2 minutes.

When the timer beeps, naturally release pressure. Open the lid with care.

Crush the cranberries with a fork or masher. Stir again. Serve warm or cold.

# Very Cheesy Cheese Sauce

**Prep + Cook Time**: 10 minutes

## Ingredients

- 2 Tablespoons ghee

- ½ cup cream cheese, softened

- 1 cup cheddar cheese, grated

- 1 cup mozzarella cheese, grated

- 2 Tablespoons water (or coconut milk)

- ½ cup heavy whipping cream

- 1 teaspoon of salt

## Directions:

Press Sauté button on Instant Pot. Melt the ghee.

Add cream cheese, cheddar cheese, mozzarella cheese, water or/coconut milk, heavy whipping cream, and salt. Stir constantly until melted.

Press Keep Warm/Cancel button to end sauté mode.

Close and seal lid. Press Manual switch. Cook at High Pressure for 4 minutes.

Quick-release or naturally release pressure when done. Open the lid with care. Stir. Serve.

# Best Homemade Alfredo Sauce

**Prep + Cook Time**: 15 minutes

## Ingredients

-       1 cup coconut milk

-       2 cups Parmesan cheese, grated

-       1 onion, chopped

-       1 teaspoon of salt

-       ½ lemon, juice

-       ¼ cup + 1 Tablespoon nutritional yeast

-       2 Tablespoons ghee

-       1 teaspoon garlic powder

-       1 teaspoon ground nutmeg

-       1 teaspoon salt

-       1 teaspoon fresh ground black pepper

## Directions:

Press Sauté button on Instant Pot. Heat the ghee.

Sauté the garlic and onion until become translucent.

Add coconut milk, parmesan cheese, nutritional yeast, lemon juice, and seasonings. Stir constantly until smooth.

Press Keep Warm/Cancel button. Cook at High Pressure for 6 minutes.

Quick-release or naturally release pressure when done. Open the lid with care. Stir. Serve.

# Knockout Asparagus and Shrimp Mix

**Prep + Cook Time**: 10 minutes

## Ingredients

- 1 pound asparagus, trimmed and chopped

- 1 pound shrimp, peeled and deveined

- 2 Tablespoons ghee, melted

- 2 cups of water

- 1 teaspoon salt (to taste)

- 1 teaspoon fresh ground black pepper (to taste)

## Directions:

Pour 2 cups of water in Instant Pot.

Place shrimp and asparagus in steamer basket. Drizzle melted ghee over shrimp and asparagus. Season with salt and pepper. Place basket in Instant Pot.

Close and seal lid. Press Manual button. Cook at High Pressure for 6 minutes.

When the timer beeps, release pressure naturally. Open the lid with care. Serve.

# Heavenly Stuffed Bell Peppers

**Prep + Cook Time**: 30 minutes

## Ingredients

- 1 pound lean ground beef

- 1 teaspoon coconut oil

- 4 medium to large bell peppers, de-seeded, tops sliced off

- 1 avocado, chopped

- Juice from 1 lime

- 1 jalapeno, minced (depending on heat level, remove or leave seeds)

- 2 green onions, chopped

- 2 cups of water

- 1 cup mixed cheeses, shredded

- 2 teaspoons chili powder

- 1 teaspoon garlic powder

- 1 teaspoon ground cumin

- 1 teaspoon salt (to taste)

- 1 teaspoon fresh ground black pepper (to taste)

## Directions:

Press Sauté button on Instant Pot. Heat the coconut oil. Sauté ground beef until no longer pink; drain.

Place ground beef in a bowl. Add green onions, jalapeno, and seasoning. Stir well.

Stuff mixture in bell peppers.

Pour 2 cups of water in Instant Pot. Place stuffed peppers in steamer basket. Top with shredded cheese.

Close and seal lid. Press Manual button. Cook at High Pressure for 15 minutes.

When done, naturally release pressure. Open the lid with care. Serve.

# Hollywood Collard Greens and Bacon

**Prep + Cook Time**: 15 minutes

## Ingredients

- 1 pound collard greens, trimmed and chopped

- ¼ pound bacon, chopped

- ½ cup ghee, melted

- 1 teaspoon salt

- 1 teaspoon fresh ground black pepper

## Directions:

Press Sauté button on Instant Pot. Melt 1 tablespoon of ghee. Add the bacon. Sauté until bacon is brown and crispy. Press Keep Warm/Cancel button to end Sauté mode.

Add collard greens, rest of the ghee, salt and pepper. Stir well.

Close and seal lid. Press Manual button. Cook at High Pressure for 10 minutes.

When done, naturally release pressure. Open the lid with care. Stir. Serve.

# Godly Kale Delish

**Prep + Cook Time**: 15 minutes

## Ingredients

-        1 bunch of kale, trimmed and chopped

-        1 red onion, thinly sliced

-        4 garlic cloves, minced

-        1 cup pine nuts, roughly chopped

-        1 cup vegetable broth

-        1 Tablespoon ghee, melted

-        2 Tablespoons coconut oil

-        1 Tablespoon balsamic vinegar

-        1 teaspoon red pepper flakes

-        1 teaspoon salt

-        1 teaspoon fresh ground black pepper

## Directions:

Press Sauté button on Instant Pot. Heat the coconut oil.

Sauté onion and garlic until translucent. Press Keep Warm/Cancel button to end Sauté mode.

Add kale, pine nuts, melted ghee, balsamic vinegar, pine nuts, red pepper flakes, salt and pepper. Stir well. Close and seal lid. Press Manual button. Cook at High Pressure for 8 minutes.

Quick-Release the pressure when done. Open the lid with care.

Adjust seasoning if needed. Serve.

# Creamy Brussel Sprouts with Garlic Cream Cheese

**Prep + Cook Time**: 10 minutes

## Ingredients

2 tablespoons of unsalted butter

2 pounds of brussel sprouts, trimmed and cut half lengthwise

5 medium garlic cloves, peeled and minced

1 ½ cup of homemade low-sodium vegetable stock or chicken stock

¾ cup of cream cheese, softened

¼ cup of parmesan cheese, grated

Fine sea salt and freshly cracked black pepper (to taste)

## Directions:

Add all the ingredients except for the parmesan inside your Instant Pot. Lock the lid and cook at high pressure for 2 minutes. When the cooking is done, quick release the pressure and carefully remove the lid. Stir in the grated parmesan cheese and cover with the lid. Sit for 5 minutes or until the sauce thickens. Give another good stir. Serve and enjoy!

# Brussel Sprouts with Cranberries and Balsamic Vinegar

**Prep + Cook Time**: 25 minutes

## Ingredients

3 pounds of brussel sprouts, trimmed and halved

½ cup of extra-virgin olive oil

1 cup of dried cranberries

¾ cups of balsamic vinegar

1 cup of water

Fine sea salt and freshly cracked black pepper (to taste)

## Directions:

Add 1 cup of water and a steamer basket inside your Instant Pot. Add the brussel sprouts in the steamer basket.

Lock the lid and cook at high pressure for 3 minutes.

When the cooking is done, quick release the pressure and remove the lid. Remove the steamer basket and discard the water.

Transfer the brussel sprouts to a baking sheet lined with aluminum foil. Add the dried cranberries. Drizzle with the cranberries, extra-virgin olive oil and balsamic vinegar. Sprinkle with sea salt and freshly cracked black pepper.

Set your oven to 370 degrees Fahrenheit. Place inside your oven and bake for around 5 minutes. Toss until well combined. Serve and enjoy!

# Spinach Crab Dip

**Prep + Cook Time**: 45 minutes

## Ingredients

4-ounces of frozen chopped spinach

3 (6-ounce) cans of crabmeat, drained

1/3 cup of homemade mayonnaise

¼ cup of full-fat coconut milk

2 tablespoons of almond flour

2 tablespoons of nutritional yeast

2 tablespoons of unsalted butter or ghee

1 medium red onion, finely chopped

3 medium garlic cloves, minced

1 teaspoon of old bay seasoning

2 green onions, finely chopped

Fine sea salt and freshly cracked black pepper (to taste)

## Directions:

Press the "Sauté" setting on your Instant Pot and add the butter. Once melted, add the chopped red onion and sauté until tender, stirring occasionally.

Add the remaining ingredients. Lock the lid and cook at high pressure for 10 minutes.

When the cooking is done, naturally release the pressure for 5 minutes, then quick release the remaining pressure. Carefully remove the lid. Serve and enjoy!

# Spaghetti Squash

**Prep + Cook Time**: 25 minutes

**Ingredients**

1 (2 pound) spaghetti squash, cut half lengthwise

1 cup of water

**Directions:**

Add 1 cup of water and a steamer basket or trivet inside your Instant Pot. Place the squash on top. Lock the lid and cook at high pressure for 7 minutes.

When the cooking is done, manually release the pressure and remove the lid.

Shred the spaghetti squash using two forks. Serve and enjoy!

# Roasted Brussel Sprouts

**Prep + Cook Time**: 20 minutes

## Ingredients

2 tablespoons of coconut oil, melted

1 pound of whole brussel sprouts, trimmed

1 medium onion, roughly chopped

½ cup of homemade low-sodium vegetable stock

Fine sea salt and freshly cracked black pepper (to taste)

## Directions:

Press the "Sauté" function on your Instant Pot and add the olive oil. Once hot, add the onions and sauté for 2 minutes or until translucent, stirring occasionally.

Add the brussel sprouts and cook for another minute. Season with sea salt and black pepper.

Pour in the vegetable stock and lock the lid. Cook at high pressure for 3 minutes. When the cooking is done, quick release the pressure and carefully remove the lid. Serve and enjoy!

# Delicious Broccoli and Garlic Combo

**Prep + Cook Time**: 15 minutes

## Ingredients

- 1 broccoli head, chopped into florets

- 2 Tablespoons coconut oil

- 6 garlic cloves, minced

- 2 cups of water

- 1 teaspoon salt (to taste)

- 1 teaspoon black pepper (to taste)

## Directions:

Press Sauté button on Instant Pot. Heat the coconut oil.

Sauté garlic for 2 minutes. Add the broccoli. Cook until softened. Set aside.

Press Keep Warm/Cancel button to end Sauté mode.

Pour 2 cups of water in Instant Pot. Place garlic and broccoli florets in steamer basket. Season with salt and black pepper.

Close and seal lid. Press Manual button. Cook at High Pressure for 10 minutes.

When done, naturally release pressure. Open the lid with care.

Transfer to a bowl. Stir well. Serve.

# Hot Dogs with a Twist

**Prep + Cook Time**: 10 minutes

## Ingredients

-       8 hot dogs

-       1 cup low-carb beer

-       8 ketogenic hot dog buns (for serving)

## Directions:

Place the hot dogs in Instant Pot. Pour beer over the hot dogs.

Close and seal the lid. Press Manual button. Cook at High Pressure for 5 minutes.

Quick-Release the pressure when done. Open the lid with care. Serve, on buns or alone.

# Perfect Marinara Sauce

**Prep + Cook Time**: 15 minutes

## Ingredients

- 2 (14-ounce) cans diced tomatoes

- 2 Tablespoons red wine vinegar

- ¼ cup coconut oil

- 1 teaspoon onion powder

- 1 teaspoon garlic powder

- 1 Tablespoon fresh oregano, chopped

- 1 Tablespoon fresh basil, chopped

- 1 Tablespoon fresh parsley, chopped

- 1 teaspoon salt

- 1 teaspoon fresh ground black pepper

## Directions:

Add the ingredients to Instant Pot. Stir well.

Close and seal lid. Press Manual button. Cook at High Pressure for 8 minutes.

When the timer beeps, naturally release pressure. Open the lid with care.

Puree mixture with immersion blender. Serve.

# Zesty Onion and Cauliflower Dip

**Prep + Cook Time**: 20 minutes

## Ingredients

- 1 head cauliflower, minced

- 1 cup chicken broth

- 1 ¼ cup low-carb mayonnaise

- 1 onion, chopped

- 1 cup cream cheese, softened

- 1 teaspoon Chili powder

- 1 teaspoon ground cumin

- 1 teaspoon garlic powder

- 1 teaspoon salt (to taste)

- 1 teaspoon fresh ground black pepper (to taste)

## Directions:

Add all ingredients to Instant Pot. Stir well. Using a hand blender, blend ingredients.

Close and seal lid. Press Manual button. Cook at High Pressure for 10 minutes.

When the timer beeps, naturally release pressure, Open the lid with care. Stir ingredients. Serve.

# Ultimate Corn on the Cob

**Prep + Cook Time**: 20 minutes

## Ingredients

- 8 corn on the cob

- 2 cups of water

- 2 teaspoons low-carb brown sugar

- 1 teaspoon salt (to taste)

- 1 teaspoon fresh ground black pepper (to taste)

## Directions:

Pour 2 cups of water in Instant Pot. Place corn in steamer basket. Place basket in Instant Pot.

Close and seal lid. Press Manual button. Cook at High Pressure for 5 minutes.

When the timer beeps, naturally release pressure. Open the lid with care.

Sprinkle with brown sugar. Serve.

# Chapter 12: Second Course Recipes (30 Recipes)

## Enticing Chicken and Broccoli Casserole

**Prep + Cook Time**: 65 minutes

**Ingredients**

1 pound of broccoli florets

3 boneless, skinless chicken breasts, cooked and cut into bite-sized pieces

3 cups of cheddar cheese, shredded or finely grated

1 cup of homemade zero-sugar mayonnaise

2 tablespoons of coconut oil, melted

½ teaspoon of freshly cracked black pepper

1/3 cup of homemade low-sodium chicken stock

½ teaspoon of sea salt

2 tablespoons of freshly squeezed lemon juice

**Directions:**

Preheat your oven to 350 degrees Fahrenheit. Grease a baking dish with the coconut oil.

Place the chicken pieces to the bottom of the baking dish.

Spread the broccoli florets on top of the chicken.

Spread half of the shredded cheddar cheese over the broccoli.

In a bowl, add the mayonnaise, chicken stock, sea salt, freshly cracked black pepper, and lemon juice. Pour this mixture over the chicken.

Sprinkle the remaining cheddar cheese over the baking dish and tightly cover the aluminum foil.

Place the baking dish inside your oven and bake for 30 minutes.

Once done, remove the baking dish from your oven and carefully remove the aluminum foil. Return the baking dish to your oven and bake for 20 minutes. Serve and enjoy!

# Italian-Inspired Chicken Breast

**Prep + Cook Time:** 30 minutes

## Ingredients

4 boneless, skinless chicken breasts

1 pound of cherry tomatoes, halved

4 garlic cloves, finely minced

¼ cup of olive oil or extra-virgin olive oil

1 medium red onion, finely chopped

½ cup of green olives, pitted and chopped

4 anchovy fillets, chopped

1 tablespoon of capers, chopped

1 teaspoon of sea salt

1 teaspoon of freshly cracked black pepper

## Directions:

Preheat your oven to 450 degrees Fahrenheit.

Season the chicken breast with sea salt and black pepper. Rub half of the olive oil with the chicken breasts.

Place a skillet over high heat. Add the chicken breast and cook for 2 minutes per side.

Transfer the chicken breasts to a baking pan.

Transfer the chicken breasts to a baking pan. Place the baking pan inside your oven and bake for 8 minutes.

Once done, transfer the chicken breasts on plates. Set aside.

Add the chopped onion, minced garlic, chopped olives, anchovies, halved cherry tomatoes and capers to the skillet. Cook for 1 minute, stirring occasionally.

Drizzle the tomato mixture over the chicken breasts.Transfer to containers and enjoy!

# Energetic Lemon Chicken

**Prep + Cook Time**: 55 minutes

**Ingredients**

6 boneless, skinless chicken breasts or chicken thighs

1 medium onion, chopped

6 garlic cloves, minced

2 tablespoons of olive oil

2 teaspoons of sea salt

2 teaspoons of freshly cracked black pepper

Juice and zest from 2 medium-sized lemons

1 lemon, cut into wedges

**Directions**:

Preheat your oven to 375 degrees Fahrenheit.

Place the chicken onto a baking dish and season with sea salt and black pepper.

Add the chopped onion, minced garlic, lemon juice, olive oil and lemon zest. Stir until well incorporated.

Add the lemon wedges.

Place the baking dish inside your oven and bake for 45 minutes or until the chicken is cooked through.

Remove the baking dish from your oven and discard the lemon wedges.

Transfer the lemon chicken to containers and enjoy!

# Excellent Creamy Chicken

**Prep + Cook Time**: 60 minutes

## Ingredients

4 boneless, skinless chicken breasts

½ cup of homemade zero-sugar mayonnaise

½ cup of organic sour cream

¾ cup of parmesan cheese, finely grated

8 slices of mozzarella cheese

1 tablespoon of olive oil

1 teaspoon of onion powder

1 teaspoon of garlic powder

1/2 teaspoon of paprika

½ teaspoon of freshly cracked black pepper

½ teaspoon of sea salt

## Directions:

Preheat your oven to 375 degrees Fahrenheit. Grease a baking dish with 1 tablespoon of olive oil.

Place the chicken breast on the baking dish.

In a bowl, mix the grated parmesan cheese, mayonnaise, sour cream, onion powder, garlic powder, paprika, sea salt, and black pepper. Mix well. Spread the mixture over the chicken.

Place the baking dish inside your oven and bake for 1 hour.

Transfer the chicken to containers and enjoy!

# Definite Pecan-Crusted Chicken

**Prep + Cook Time**: 30 minutes

## Ingredients

1 ½ cups of pecans, chopped

4 boneless, skinless chicken breasts

1 teaspoon of sea salt

1 large egg

1 teaspoon of freshly cracked black pepper

3 tablespoons of coconut oil

## Directions:

Preheat your oven to 350 degrees Fahrenheit. Line a baking sheet with parchment paper.

In a bowl, add the chopped pecans eggs. Mix well.

Season each chicken breast with sea salt and black pepper.

Heat the coconut oil in a medium skillet over medium-high heat.

Once the coconut oil is hot, add the chicken breast and cook for 4 minutes per side or until brown.

Transfer the chicken to the baking sheet and place inside your oven. Bake for 10 minutes.

Transfer to containers and enjoy!

# Flavorsome Pulled Pork

**Prep + Cook Time**: 45 minutes

## Ingredients

- 3 pounds boneless pork shoulder

- 2 Tablespoons coconut oil

- 1 teaspoon onion powder

- 1 teaspoon garlic powder

- 1 Tablespoon paprika

- 1 cup beef broth

- 1 teaspoon salt (to taste)

- 1 teaspoon fresh ground black pepper (to taste)

**Barbeque Sauce Ingredients:**

- 3 Tablespoons low-sugar ketchup

- 4 Tablespoons granulated Splenda

- ¼ cup yellow mustard

- 2 teaspoons hot sauce

- 3 Tablespoons apple cider vinegar

**Directions:**

In a small bowl, combine onion powder, garlic powder, paprika, salt and pepper. Mix well. Rub seasoning on pork shoulder.

Press Sauté mode on Instant Pot. Heat coconut oil. Sear all sides of pork shoulder.

In another bowl, combine barbecue sauce ingredients. Stir well.

Press Keep Warm/Cancel setting to end Sauté mode.

Add the barbecue sauce and beef broth to Instant Pot. Stir well.

Close and seal lid. Press Manual button. Cook on high pressure for 35 minutes.

Quick-release or naturally release pressure when done. Open the lid with care.

Use two forks to pull pork apart.

Press Sauté button. Simmer until sauce reduced and clings to pork.

Press Keep Warm/Cancel button. Serve.

# Hearty Lemon & Garlic Pork

**Prep + Cook Time**: 25 minutes

## Ingredients

- 4 pork chops, boneless

- 2 cups beef broth

- 3 Tablespoons ghee, melted

- 3 Tablespoons coconut oil

- 1 teaspoon salt

- 1 teaspoon fresh ground black pepper

- Zest and juice from 2 lemons

- 6 garlic cloves, minced

- ¼ cup fresh parsley, chopped

## Directions:

Season the pork chops with salt and pepper, lemon juice and zest.

Press the Sauté button on your Instant Pot. Heat coconut oil.

Sauté garlic for 1 minute. Add pork chops. Sear for 2 minutes per side.

Press the Keep Warm/Cancel button to end Sauté mode.Add ghee and beef broth to the Instant Pot. Close and seal lid. Press Poultry button. Cook for 15 minutes.

Quick-release pressure when done. Open the lid with care. Stir ingredients. Serve.

# Tasty Thai Beef

**Prep + Cook Time**: 30 minutes

## Ingredients

- 1 pound of beef, cut into strips

- 1 green bell pepper, chopped

- 1 red bell pepper, chopped

- Zest and juice from 1 lemon

- 2 cups beef broth

- 2 teaspoons ginger, grated

- 4 garlic cloves, minced

- 2 Tablespoons coconut oil

- 1 Tablespoon coconut amino

- 1 cup roasted pecans

- 1 teaspoon salt

- 1 teaspoon fresh ground black pepper

## Directions:

Press Sauté button on Instant Pot. Heat the coconut oil.

Sauté garlic and ginger for 1 minute. Add beef strips. Sear 1-2 minutes per side.

Add bell peppers. Add salt and pepper.

Continue cooking until meat is no longer pink.

Add coconut amino, pecans, zest and juice from lemon, beef broth. Stir well.

Close and seal lid. Press Manual setting. Cook at High Pressure for 15 minutes.

Release pressure naturally when done. Open the lid with care. Let it sit for 5 – 10 minutes. Serve.

# Gratifying Meatloaf

**Prep + Cook Time**: 35 minutes

## Ingredients

-       3 pounds lean ground beef

-       4 garlic cloves, minced

-       1 yellow onion, chopped

-       1 cup mushrooms, chopped

-       3 large eggs

-       ½ cup almond flour

-       ¼ cup parmesan cheese, grated

-       ¼ cup mozzarella cheese, grated

-       ¼ cup fresh parsley, chopped

-       2 Tablespoons sugar-free ketchup

-       2 Tablespoons coconut oil

-       2 teaspoons salt

-       2 teaspoons black pepper

-       2 cups of water

## Directions:

Cover trivet with aluminum foil.

In a large bowl, add and mix all the ingredients (excluding the water) until well combined. Form into a meatloaf. Pour the water in your Instant Pot. Place trivet inside.

Place meatloaf on trivet.

Close and seal lid. Press Manual button. Cook at High-Pressure for 25 minutes.

Release pressure naturally when done.. Open the lid with care.

Let the meatloaf rest for 5 minutes before slicing and serve.

# Lavender Lamb Chops

**Prep + Cook Time**: 25 minutes

## Ingredients

-       2 lamb chops, boneless

-       2 Tablespoons ghee, melted

-       1 Tablespoon lavender, chopped

-       2 Tablespoons coconut oil

-       2 Tablespoons fresh rosemary, chopped

-       Zest and juice from 1 orange

-       Zest and juice from 1 lime

-       1 teaspoon garlic powder

-       1 teaspoon salt

-       1 teaspoon fresh ground black pepper

-       2 cups of water

## Directions:

Cover trivet with aluminum foil.

Press Sauté button on Instant Pot. Heat the coconut oil.

Sear lamb chops for 2 minutes per side. Remove and set aside.

Press Keep Warm/Cancel button to end Sauté mode.

In a bowl, add and mix the ghee, lavender, rosemary, orange juice, orange zest, lime juice, lime zest, and seasonings.

Pour 2 cups of water in Instant Pot. Place trivet inside. Set lamb chops on top.

Close and seal lid. Press Manual button. Cook at High Pressure for 15 minutes.

Quick-release the pressure when done. Open the lid with care. Serve.

# Flavorful Avocado Lime Halibut

**Prep + Cook Time**: 30 minutes

## Ingredients

2 (6-ounces) of boneless halibut fillets or any other fish

1 large head of cauliflower, chopped

2 large avocados

2 tablespoons of freshly squeezed lime juice

¼ cup of red onions, finely chopped

2 tablespoons of olive oil or any other cooking fat

¼ teaspoon of sea salt

¼ teaspoon of freshly cracked black pepper

## Directions:

In a food processor, add the cauliflower and pulse until rice consistency.

Grease a medium-sized skillet with 1 tablespoon of olive oil over medium heat.

Add the rice cauliflower and cook for 8 minutes or until tender. Remove and set aside.

Clean out your food processor and add the avocados, lime juice, and red onions. Blend until smooth.

Heat the remaining tablespoon of olive oil in a large skillet over medium-high heat.

Season the fish fillets with sea salt and black pepper. You can add any other spices if you prefer.

Working in batches, if necessary, add the fish fillets and cook for 4 to 5 minutes per side.

Serve and enjoy along with the cauliflower rice and drizzle of the avocado mixture.

# Awesome Tuna Egg Casserole

**Prep + Cook Time**: 20 minutes

## Ingredients

2 to 3 cans of tuna

1 (14.5-ounce) can of artichoke hearts, drained and chopped

6 cups of arugula greens

6 eggs

½ teaspoon of freshly cracked black pepper

½ cup of cheddar cheese or mozzarella cheese, shredded

½ teaspoon of sea salt

## Directions:

Preheat your oven to 375 degrees Fahrenheit. In a large bowl, combine the tuna and artichoke hearts.

Transfer the tuna mixture to a greased baking dish.

Crack the eggs over the tuna mixture and lightly sprinkle with cheddar cheese, sea salt, and black pepper.

Place the dish inside your oven and bake for 10 minutes.

Carefully remove the dish from your oven and allow to cool.

Place the arugula into a bowl and add the tuna mixture over the arugula greens. Transfer to containers and enjoy!

# Herbed Salmon Fillets

**Prep + Cook Time**: 25 minutes

## Ingredients

4 (6-ounce) boneless salmon fillets

1 tablespoon of fresh parsley, chopped

1 tablespoon of fresh basil, chopped

1 tablespoon of fresh thyme, chopped

4 fresh rosemary sprig

4 whole garlic cloves

½ teaspoon of freshly cracked black pepper

2 tablespoons of olive oil

½ teaspoon of sea salt

½ teaspoon of onion powder

2 lemons, sliced

## Directions:

Preheat your oven to 390 degrees Fahrenheit.

In a bowl, add the fresh parsley, fresh basil, fresh thyme, olive oil, sea salt, black pepper, and onion powder. Mix until well combined. Grease a baking sheet and place the salmon fillets on top.

Add the herbed mixture over the salmon and gently place lemon slices, rosemary sprig, and whole garlic cloves on top. Place inside your oven and bake for 10 to 13 minutes or until cooked through.

Serve and enjoy!

# Timely Chipotle Fish Tacos

**Prep + Cook Time**: 15 minutes

## Ingredients

2 tablespoons of olive oil

2 tablespoons of butter or coconut oil

1 pound of salmon, tilapia, sea bass or haddock fish fillets

2 garlic cloves, crushed

2 tablespoons of keto-friendly sugar-free mayonnaise

2 tablespoons of butter

1 medium-sized yellow onion, finely chopped

1 medium-sized jalapeno pepper, finely sliced

2 chipotle peppers in adobo sauce, minced

4 low-carb (preferably homemade) tortillas or lettuce wraps

## Directions:

In a medium skillet, heat 2 tablespoons of coconut oil over high-heat.

Once the olive oil is hot, add the onions and cook for 5 minutes or until translucent, stirring occasionally.

Lower the heat and add in the crushed garlic and sliced jalapeno peppers. Cook for 2 minutes, stirring occasionally. Mince the chipotle peppers and stir them in with the adobo sauce.

Add the fish fillets to the skillet along with the mayonnaise and butter.

Stir everything together and cook for 8 minutes or until the fish is cooked.

To make the tacos: Fill tortillas with the fish mixture and store in containers.

# Spicy Spirited Lemon Salmon

**Prep + Cook Time**: 20 minutes

## Ingredients

- 4 salmon fillets

- Juice from 2 lemons + slices for garnish

- 1 cup of water

- 1 Tablespoon paprika

- 1 teaspoon cayenne pepper

- 1 teaspoon salt (to taste)

- 1 teaspoon fresh ground black pepper (to taste)

## Directions:

Rinse the salmon, pat dry.

In a bowl, combine salt, pepper, paprika, cayenne pepper.

Drizzle lemon juice over salmon fillet. Season with spice mixture. Turn over fillet, repeat on other side.

Add 1 cup of water to Instant Pot. Place trivet inside. Place fillets on trivet.

Close and seal cover. Press Manual button. Cook at High Pressure for 10 minutes.

Quick-Release the pressure when done. Open the lid with care. Serve.

# Awesome Coconut Shrimp Curry

**Prep + Cook Time**: 35 minutes

## Ingredients

- 1 pound shrimp, peeled and deveined

- 1 Tablespoon coconut oil

- 4 garlic cloves, minced

- Juice from 1 lime

- 1 teaspoon salt

- 1 teaspoon fresh ground black pepper

- 4 tomatoes, chopped

- 1 red bell pepper, sliced

- 10-ounces coconut milk

- ½ cup fresh cilantro, chopped

## Directions:

Press Sauté mode on Instant Pot. Heat the coconut oil.

Season shrimp with lime juice, salt and pepper. Sauté garlic for 1 minute.

Add shrimp. Cook 2 – 4 minutes per side. Add bell peppers and tomatoes. Stir well.

Press Keep Warm/Cancel button to cancel Sauté mode. Add coconut milk. Stir well.

Close and seal lid. Press Manual setting. Cook at High Pressure for 25 minutes.

Quick-Release the pressure when done. Open the lid with care. Garnish with fresh cilantro. Serve.

# Wild Alaskan Cod

**Prep + Cook Time**: 25 minutes

## Ingredients

- 4 wild Alaskan cod fillets

- 4 cups cherry tomatoes, halved

- 4 garlic cloves, minced

- 4 Tablespoons butter, melted

- 1 Tablespoon coconut oil

- ¼ cup of fresh cilantro, chopped

- 1 teaspoon salt (to taste)

- 1 teaspoon fresh ground black pepper (to taste)

## Directions:

On a flat surface, rub garlic over cod fillets. Season with salt and pepper.

Cover trivet with foil. Add 1 cup of water to Instant Pot. Place trivet inside.

Place tomatoes along bottom of Instant Pot. Season with salt and pepper.

Place salmon fillets on trivet.

Pour melted butter and coconut oil over cod fillets and tomatoes.

Close and seal lid. Press Manual switch. Cook at High Pressure for 15 minutes.

When the timer beeps, quick-release pressure. Open the lid with care.

Plate the fillets. Top with tomatoes and fresh cilantro. Serve.

# Stunning Shrimp and Sausage Gumbo

**Prep + Cook Time**: 35 minutes

## Ingredients

- 1 pound shrimp, peeled and deveined

- 1 pound lean sausage, thinly sliced

- 1 red bell pepper, chopped

- 1 yellow onion, chopped

- 1 garlic clove, minced

- 1 celery stalk, chopped

- 2 cups chicken broth

- ½ cup fresh parsley, chopped

- 2 Tablespoons coconut oil

- 2 Tablespoons Cajun seasoning

- 1 teaspoon salt (to taste)

- 1 teaspoon fresh ground black pepper (to taste)

## Directions:

Press Sauté button on Instant Pot. Heat the coconut oil.

Sauté onion and garlic for 1 minute.

Add sausage and shrimp. Cook until golden brown.

Add bell pepper and celery. Season with Cajun spice. Stir well.

Press Keep Warm/Cancel setting to stop Sauté mode.

Add 2 cups of chicken broth. Stir well.

Close and seal lid. Press Meat/Stew button. Adjust to cook for 25 minutes.

When the timer beeps, quick-release or naturally release pressure. Open the lid with care. Stir well. Serve.

# Wondrous Mediterranean Fish

**Prep + Cook Time**: 25 minutes

## Ingredients

- 4 fish fillets (any kind)

- 1 pound cherry tomatoes, halved

- 1 cup green olives, pitted

- 2 garlic cloves, minced

- 1 cup of water

- 1 teaspoon coconut oil

- 1 Tablespoon fresh thyme, chopped

- 1 teaspoon fresh parsley

- 1 teaspoon salt (to taste)

- 1 teaspoon fresh ground black pepper (to taste)

## Directions:

Pour 1 cup of water in Instant Pot. Cover trivet in foil.

On a flat surface, rub fish fillets with garlic. Season with salt, pepper and thyme.

Place olives and cherry tomatoes along bottom of Instant Pot. Place fillets on trivet.

Close and seal lid. Press Manual button. Cook at High Pressure for 15 minutes.

Release pressure naturally when done. Open the lid with care.

Place the fish with the ingredients. Stir to coat them.

Plate the fillets. Top with fresh parsley. Serve.

# Incredible Tilapia with Tomato and Avocado Salad

**Prep + Cook Time**: 30 minutes

**Ingredients**

8 (6-ounce) tilapia fillets

5 tablespoons of coconut oil

½ teaspoon of freshly cracked black pepper (more to taste)

2 tablespoons of plain Greek yogurt

2 garlic cloves, minced

½ teaspoon of sea salt (more to taste)

4 tablespoons of freshly squeezed lemon juice

2 tablespoons of fresh lemon zest

1 teaspoon of dried oregano

1 cups of avocados, diced

1 cups of cherry tomatoes, halved

**Directions:**

In a bowl, combine the lemon juice, lemon zest, plain Greek yogurt, minced garlic, sea salt and black pepper.

Add 4 tablespoons of coconut oil. Stir until well combined.

In a large Ziploc bag, add the tilapia fillets along with the yogurt mixture.

Place the bag inside your refrigerator and allow to marinate for 20 minute or overnight.

Preheat your oven to 400 degrees Fahrenheit. Place the tilapia fillets on a baking dish and place inside your oven.

Bake for 10 to 12 minutes or until the tilapia fillets are cooked through.

In a bowl, add the diced avocados, halved cherry tomatoes, and 1 tablespoon of coconut oil.

Place 1 tilapia fillets per ½ cup of salad and transfer to containers. Serve and enjoy!

# Greek-Inspired Salmon Salad

**Prep + Cook Time**: 30 minutes

## Ingredients

2 pounds of boneless salmon fillets

½ teaspoon of freshly cracked black pepper

1 head of romaine lettuce, chopped

1 medium-sized cucumber, chopped

½ teaspoon of sea salt

2 tablespoons of fresh chives, chopped

6-ounces of feta cheese

1 tablespoon of oregano

½ cup of extra-virgin olive oil

3 tablespoons of freshly squeezed lime juice or lemon juice

¾ cups of Kalamata olives, roughly chopped

## Directions:

Preheat your oven to 450 degrees Fahrenheit. Drizzle 2 tablespoons of salmon over the salmon fillets.

Season the salmon with sea salt and black pepper. Transfer to a baking dish.

Place the dish inside your oven and bake for 15 minutes.

Once done, remove from your oven and cut into bite-sized pieces

In a large bowl, add the salmon and remaining ingredients except for the olive oil. Stir until everything is well coated. Transfer the salad to containers and reserve the olive oil for when ready to serve. Serve and enjoy!

# Grandmother's Coconut Shrimp Soup

**Prep + Cook Time**: 30 minutes

**Ingredients**

1 pound of shrimp, peeled and deveined

1 tablespoon of freshly squeezed lime juice

1 (14-ounce) can of Thai coconut milk

1 tablespoon of coconut oil, melted

1 medium red onion, finely chopped

4 garlic cloves, minced

3 cups of homemade low-sodium fish stock

1 tablespoon of fish sauce

1 tablespoon of fresh basil

½ teaspoon of freshly cracked black pepper (more to taste)

1 teaspoon of fresh ginger, grated

2 tablespoons of fresh cilantro, finely chopped

½ teaspoon of sea salt (more to taste)

**Directions:**

In a large cooking pot, heat the coconut oil over medium-high heat.

Add the chopped red onion and minced garlic. Cook for 6 minutes or until softened, stirring occasionally.

Add the shrimp and cook until pink, stirring occasionally.

Gently stir in the remaining ingredients and bring to a boil.

Once it comes to a boil, lower the heat. Allow to simmer for around 15 minutes, stirring occasionally and adjusting the seasoning to your liking. Transfer the soup to containers and enjoy!

# Scrumptious Shrimp and Arugula Salad

**Prep + Cook Time**: 15 minutes

## Ingredients

16 cups of fresh arugula

2 pounds of shrimp, cooked and peeled

2 medium-sized avocados, peeled and diced

8 tablespoons of extra-virgin olive oil

¼ teaspoon of freshly cracked black pepper

4 medium-sized lemons, juiced

½ teaspoon of sea salt

## Directions:

In a large bowl, add the arugula, shrimp, and avocados. Stir until fully combined.

In a second bowl, add the olive oil, lemon juice, sea salt and freshly cracked black pepper. Mix well.

Store the salad into mason jars or other containers. Set the olive oil mixture aside until ready to use.

# Flavorful Beef and Tomato Stuffed Squash

**Prep + Cook Time**: 30 minutes

**Ingredients**

- 1 pound of beef, chopped into chunks

- 1 pound butternut squash, peeled and chopped

- 2 Tablespoons coconut oil

- 2 Tablespoons ghee, melted

- 1 green bell pepper, chopped

- 1 yellow bell pepper, chopped

- 2 (14-ounce) cans diced tomatoes

- 4 garlic cloves, minced

- 1 yellow or red onion, chopped

- 1 Tablespoon fresh thyme, chopped

- 1 Tablespoon fresh rosemary, chopped

- 2 Tablespoons fresh parsley, chopped

- 1 teaspoon cayenne pepper

- 1 teaspoon salt

- 1 teaspoon fresh ground black pepper

## Directions:

Press Sauté button on Instant Pot. Heat the coconut oil.

Add onion and garlic. Sweat for 2 minutes.

Add beef chunks, butternut squash, and bell peppers.

Sauté until meat is no longer pink and vegetables have softened.

Press Keep Warm/Cancel button to end Sauté mode.

Add melted ghee, tomatoes, thyme, rosemary, parsley, cayenne pepper, salt and pepper. Stir well. Close and seal lid. Press Manual button. Cook at High Pressure for 20 minutes.

Quick-release the pressure when done.. Open the lid with care. Stir ingredients. Adjust the seasoning if needed. Serve.

# Super Yummy Pork Chops

**Prep + Cook Time**: 25 minutes

## Ingredients

- 4 boneless pork chops

- 2 Tablespoons coconut oil

- 2 cups beef broth

- 4 garlic cloves, minced

- 1 teaspoon nutmeg

- 1 teaspoon paprika

- 1 teaspoon onion powder

- 1 teaspoon salt

- 1 teaspoon fresh ground black pepper

## Directions:

Season the pork chops with spices listed. Press Sauté button on Instant Pot. Heat the coconut oil. Sear pork chops for 2 minutes per side.

Press Keep Warm/Cancel button to end Sauté mode. Pour in beef broth.

Close and seal lid. Press Poultry button on control panel. Cook for 15 minutes.

Quick-release the pressure when done. Open the lid with care. Serve.

# Proud Bacon-Wrapped Chicken

**Prep + Cook Time**: 45 minutes

## Ingredients

2 pounds of boneless, skinless chicken breasts

8-ouncse of cream cheese

12 medium-sized bacon slices

1 teaspoon of sea salt

1 teaspoon of freshly cracked black pepper

1 tablespoon of fresh chives

## Directions:

Preheat your oven to 375 degrees Fahrenheit

Heat a medium frying pan over medium heat.

Add the bacon and cook until halfway cooked. Transfer the bacon to a plate lined with paper towels.

In a bowl, add the cream cheese, chives, sea salt, and black pepper. Stir until well combined.

Flatten the chicken breasts with a meat mallet and spread the cream cheese mixture evenly.

Roll the chicken breast and wrap with bacon slice.

Place the chicken breasts onto a greased baking dish and place inside your oven.

Bake for 30 minutes or until the chicken is cooked through.

Transfer the chicken to containers and enjoy!

# Creamy Chicken Soup

**Prep + Cook Time**: 30 minutes

**Ingredients**

4 cups of chicken stock

2 cups of shredded cooked chicken

4-ounces of cream cheese

3 tablespoons of butter

1 teaspoon of sea salt

1 teaspoon of freshly cracked black pepper

½ cup of sour cream

½ cup of celery, chopped

**Directions:**

In a blender, add the chicken stock, cream cheese, butter, sea salt, black pepper, and sour cream. Blend until well combined. Transfer the mixture to a large pot over medium heat. Add the celery, carrots and shredded chicken.

Allow to simmer for a couple of minutes. Transfer to bowls and enjoy!

# Captivating Salsa Chicken

**Prep + Cook Time**: 60 minutes

**Ingredients**

6 boneless, skinless chicken breasts

2 cups of jarred salsa

1 cup of cheddar cheese, shredded

1 teaspoon of freshly cracked black pepper

1 tablespoon of olive oil

1 teaspoon of sea salt

**Directions:**

Preheat your oven to 400 degrees Fahrenheit. Grease a baking dish with 1 tablespoon of olive oil.

Season the chicken breasts with sea salt and black pepper.

Place the chicken breasts onto a baking dish and pour the jarred salsa over.

Place the baking dish inside your oven and bake for 1 hour or until cooked through.

Carefully remove the baking dish from your oven and spread the shredded cheddar cheese over the chicken.

Place inside your oven and bake for 15 minutes. Transfer to containers and enjoy!

# Chapter 13: Desserts Recipes (20 Recipes)

## Pumpkin Muffins with Cream Cheese Filling

**Prep + Cook Time**: 40 minutes

**Ingredients**

Filling

160 g cream cheese, softened

2½ tbsp erythritol powder

1 tsp heavy cream

½ tsp vanilla extract

Muffins

2 cups almond flour

½ cup erythritol powder

¼ cup unflavored whey powder

2 tsp baking powder

2 tsp pumpkin pie spice

Pinch of salt

2 eggs

55 g pumpkin puree

55 g butter, melted

¼ cup unsweetened almond milk

½ tsp vanilla extract

## Directions

1. Mix the cream cheese and ingredients together till it turns to smooth batter.

2. Whisk the almond flour, protein powder, baking powder, pumpkin pie spice, sweetener, and salt in a medium bowl. Preheat the oven to 320°F (160°C) and line the muffin tin with paper liners or use silicone.

3. Mix the pumpkin puree, eggs, melt butter, almond milk and vanilla extract until incorporated.

4. Add a spoonful batter into each muffin well. And then, create a dent for cream cheese, filling in the muffins. To the center of each muffin add spoonful of filling, then top the muffins with a little more of batter.

5. Bake for 25 minutes, or until the muffins are cooked in the middle. Leave the muffins to cool before removing from the tray.

# Strawberry Shortcake

**Prep + Cook Time**: 20 minutes

## Ingredients

2 strawberries

2tbsp butter, divided, melted

2 large eggs, divided

½ tsp stevia glycerite

¼ tsp vanilla extract

1½ tbsp coconut flour

½ tbsp almond flour

½ tsp baking powder

¼ cup heavy cream

¼ teaspoon stevia glycerite

⅛ teaspoon vanilla extract

## Directions

1. Wash and dry the strawberries. Slice them to make the fine slices. Leave your strawberries to the room temperature in a small bowl.

2. For each of 2 cakes, using a fork, mix 1 tablespoon coconut flour, 1/4 teaspoon baking powder, 1/4 teaspoon stevia glycerite, 1/8 teaspoon vanilla extract, 1 tablespoon melted butter and 1 large egg, in a small microwavable bowl (my bowls are 2 inches on the bottom and 4 inches at the top)

3. On high, microwave each cake for 1 minute and 30seconds, till it puffed and set.

4. Gently loosen the cakes' edges from the bowls onto a plate with a small knife, then slice crosswise into 2 slice: the bottom one thicker, and another top thinner.

5. Whisk the heaver cream, 1/4 teaspoon stevia glycerite and 1/8 teaspoon vanilla extract in a small mixer bowl, whisking on high speed about 1 minute until the cream turns into fluffy whipped cream.

6. Top the bottom layer with half-sliced strawberries and whipped cream, then top it with the other slice for each cake... Ready for serve.

# Strawberry Pancakes

**Prep + Cook Time**: 15 minutes

## Ingredients

30 eggs

1/4 cup almond flour

1/2 ground vanilla bean

1 tbsp erythritol

1/4 tsp baking soda

1/2 tsp cream of tartar

1/4 tsp cinnamon

50 ml unsweetened coconut milk

3 ½ tbsp heavy cream

2 strawberries, chopped

salt

Some butter for fry

## Directions

1. Add all the ingredients in a bowl. Using a whisk, mix thoroughly. Let the batter sit for about 5 minutes to thicken slightly.

2. Add butter to a frying pan. Heat until almost smoking. Once it hot, turn to a low heat and wait for 30 seconds.

3. Spoon the mixture into the pan on a low heat, forming approx. 3 pancakes with 10cm in diameter then flip when golden brown

# Keto Cinnamon Donuts

**Prep + Cook Time**: 30 minutes

**Ingredients**

For Donut

200 g sour cream

60 g heavy whipping cream

4 eggs

1 tsp vanilla extract

½ cup coconut flour

¼ tsp nutmeg

¼ tsp baking soda

¼ cup erythritol powder

½ tsp salt

For Cinnamon Coating

¼ cup erythritol powder

1 tsp Cinnamon

For Cooking

60 ml coconut oil

## Directions

1. Preheat the oven to 180 degree Celcius (355°F).

2. Mix together the sour cream, whipping cream, vanilla extract and eggs in a large bowl.

3. Gently add the dry ingredients into the wet ingredients and thoroughly combined.

4. Using a donut pan or a muffin tin with scrunched up baking paper in the middle. Gently pour the batter to ¾ fill the mould suitably, and place in the oven until fix to touch on the outside (10-15 minutes).

5. Take away the donuts and let cool.

6. Fill the coconut oil in a frying pan, heat up and fry each donut for around 2 minutes each side or until golden brown.

7. Place the cinnamon and erythritol together on a plate, and roll the donuts in the compound.

# Lemon Curd

**Prep + Cook Time**: 20 minutes

## Ingredients

4 lemons for juice and zest

½ cup erythritol

½ cup Butter

3 eggs

1 egg yolk

## Directions

1. Choose a medium heatproof bowl and squeeze the lemons, zest the skin, add the butter and erythritol. Set the bowl over a pan of lightly simmering water and don't let the bowl touch the bottom of the pan. Whisk together the mixture until all the butter has melted.

2. Softly whisk the eggs and egg yolk and stir into the heated compound. Stir and cook for about 10 minutes until the compound cover the back of a spoon.

3. Take away from the heat and put the compound into sterilised jars.

Store in the refrigerator for 2 weeks or more.

# Raspberry Mousse

**Prep + Cook Time**: 40 minutes

## Ingredients

120 g fresh raspberries

4 tbs xylitol sweetener

½ cup cold water

2 tsp unflavored gelatin powder

4 tbs boiling water

1 cup heavy cream

mint leaves for decoration (optional)

## Directions

1. Add the raspberries, cold water and sweetener to a small saucepan, and heat **over a low temperature until the raspberries are fully soft and** falling apart.

2. Push the compound through a fine sieve and set aside to cool.

3. Add the gelatin and the boiling water to a small bowl and whisk until completely dissolved, then whisk it into the raspberry mixture.

4. Stir the heavy cream in a stand mixer until it becomes super soft.

5. Wrap the raspberry mixture into the cream and spoon into serving glasses or bowls.

6. Cover and leave in the refrigerator until needed.

# Brownie

**Prep + Cook Time**: 60 minutes

## Ingredients

140 g unsalted butter

160 g xylitol powdered

100 g cocoa powder

1/2 tbs salt

2 eggs at room temperature

80 g almond flour

## Directions

1. Add cocoa powder, salt, sweetener, and butter into a medium heat-proof bowl. Melt over a water bath, whisking steadily. Heat up till the sweetener has melt and the mixture is combined. Remove the mixture from the heat and let it slightly cool.

2. Whisk an egg well before add more, adding one egg at a time, until completely mixed. The texture should look smooth, and sweetener merges into the mixture. .Make sure not to over-whisk. If it is over-whisk, your brownies could end up spongier rather than fudgy.

3. Add the almond flour, and whisk vigorously till completely blended (about one minute).

4. Put a rack in the lower third of the oven and preheat to 350°F (180°C). Line the bottom and sides of an 8x8-inch baking pan with parchment paper, and set aside.

5. Bake for 20-25 minutes, or until the center is just set and the inserted toothpick comes out moist. Each oven maybe different, so give a check from 15 minutes the first time.

6. Lift the brownies by the edges of the parchment paper and cut into your desired size. For getting more special clean edges, chill your brownies in a freezer for 10 minutes before cutting.

# Keto Blueberry Cake

**Prep + Cook Time**: 70 minutes

**Ingredients**

½ tbsp unsalted butter for pan

4 eggs

100 g fresh blueberries

2 tbsp whole milk

4 tbsp unsalted butter,melted, divided

1 tbsp vanilla extract

1 ½ tsp stevia glycerite

A pinch of salt

1 ½ cups blanched finely ground almond flour

½ tsp baking soda

Directions

1. Mix milk, the eggs, melted butter, vanilla stevia and kosher salt in a middle bowl.

2. Add the almond flour and whisk it until creamy. Whisk in the baking soda

3. Gently use a rubber spatula to fold 1/2 cup of blueberries into the butter

4. Pour the butter to the prepared pan and use a spatula to spread it evenly

5. Scatter the leftover blueberries on the top of cake evenly and gently press them in with your hands.

6. Preheat the oven to 350°F (175°C). Grease a 9-inch glass pie plate with half tablespoon butter.

7. Bake the cake for 30 minutes, waiting until it turns golden and smells fragrant, and a toothpick inserted in the center comes out dry.

8. Remove the pan from the oven. To chill the cake, leave it on a wire for around 20 minutes before slicing and serving.

# Keto Pumpkin Pie

**Prep + Cook Time**: 2 hours 50 minutes

## Ingredients

1 tsp coconut oil for the pan

15 g coconut flour

3 large eggs

420 g (1 can) pure pumpkin puree, unsweetened

1 ½ tsp stevia glycerite

1 tbsp pumpkin pie spice

1 tbsp vanilla extract

1 cup coconut milk, full-fat, unsweetened

## Directions

1. Lightly whisk the eggs in a medium bowl, using the hand whisk. Add the pumpkin, pumpkin pie spice, stevia, and vanilla. Then, whisk until well combined.

2. Shake well before opening the coconut milk can. Stir it thoroughly and measure 1 cup (make sure that it's smooth and lump free) and pour it into the pumpkin mixture and whisk it till incorporated. Then whisk in the coconut flour.

3. Preheat the oven to 350°F (175°C). Lubricate a 9-inch glass pie plate with coconut oil.

4. Pour the mixture to the prepared plate, using a rubber spatula. Bake it until the center looks set (with just the small jiggle) and an inserted toothpick comes out just a little moist, yet butter free. My oven takes about 40 – 45 minutes

5. Leave the pie on cooling wire for 2 hours for cooling. Then, wrap with plastic, and chill it in refrigerator at least 2 hours before slicing and serve.

6. Before serving keto crustless pumpkin pie, to release it from the pan, carefully run the knife along the edge of the pie. Use a sharp knife to slice the pie and make sure firmly slide a cake server underneath each slice before lifting. Carefully when lift your pie up, as it is fragile.

# Salty Dark Chocolate Treat

**Prep + Cook Time**: 20 minutes

## Ingredients

150 g 75% Cocoa dark chocolate bar

15pecans

2 tbsp roasted coconut flakes

1 tbsp pumpkin seeds

1 tbsp almond, sliced

some salt

## Directions

1. Melt the chocolate for 20 second intervals in the microwave oven or in a double boiler.

2. Bring out 10 small cupcake liners which are no bigger than 2 inches in diameter.

3. Add the chocolate to the cupcake liners.

4. Add coconut chips, nuts, seeds and a few salt flakes (if you like the saltier flavour) at last.

5. Store in the refrigerator and let cool.

# Keto Chocolate Chip Cookies

**Prep + Cook Time**: 50 minutes

## Ingredients

110 g almond flour

2 tbsp coconut flour

1 tbsp konjac powder

100 g 85% Cocaodark chocolate bar

1½ tsp salt

½ tsp baking soda

½tsp xanthan gum

150 g unsalted butter

120 g golden erythritol

1 tsp vanilla extract

1 egg

80 g pecans roughly chopped

## Directions

1. Add coconut flour, almond flour, konjac powder, baking soda, salt, and xanthan gum to a medium bowl. Mix until combined.

2. In a large bowl, cream butter with a mixer until softened, then add sweetener and cream till light and fluffy.

3. Add egg and Vanilla extract, and mix until just combined. With mixer on low, add in half of flour mixture-mixing till incorporated. Mix the rest.

4. Fold in pecan bits and chocolate, then wrap with cling film and put it in refrigerator for an hour.

5. Preheat the oven to 350°F (175°C) and line the baking tray with parchment paper.

6. Divide cookie dough into 18 pieces.

7. Place cookie dough on the tray. Bake for 9 – 10 minutes for small size and 12 – 13 minutes for jumbo size. Then half way through, turning the tray around 180°. To cool the cookies, leave them for 30 minutes...then ENJOY!!

# Apricot prune bread

**Total time:** 3 hours 10 minutes

**Servings:** 8

**Ingredients:**

1 egg

4/5 cup whole milk

¼ cup apricot juice

¼ cup butter

1/5 cup sugar

4 cups almond flour

1 tablespoon instant yeast

¼ teaspoon salt

5/8 cup prunes, chopped

5/8 cup dried apricots, chopped

## Directions

Add all of the ingredients to your bread machine, carefully following the instructions of the manufacturer (except apricots and prunes).

Set the program of your bread machine to BASIC/SWEET and set crust type to LIGHT or MEDIUM.

Press START.

Once the machine beeps, add apricots and prunes.

Wait until the cycle completes.

Once the loaf is ready, take the bucket out and let the loaf cool for 5 minutes.

Gently shake the bucket to remove loaf.

Transfer to a cooling rack, slice and serve.

Enjoy!

# Bread with Turkey and Raisins

**Total time:** 3 hours 10 minutes

**Servings:** 8

**Ingredients:**

20 oz turkey

1 cup of raisins

2 big onions

2 cloves chopped garlic

1 cup of milk

25 oz almond flour

10 oz rye flour

3 teaspoons dry yeast

1 egg

3 tablespoons sunflower oil

1 teaspoon sugar

Himalayan salt

**Directions**

Soak the raisins in the warm water for 10 minutes.

Boil the turkey meat with the salt on medium heat until soft. You can use the turkey breast or fillet.

Blend the cooked and soft turkey meat using a food processor until it has a smooth consistency.

Chop the onions and garlic and then fry them until clear and caramelized.

Combine the yeast with the warm water, mixing until smooth consistency.

Combine all the ingredients with the yeast, turkey, onions, raisins, garlic and then mix and knead well.

Pour some oil into a bread machine and place the dough into the bread maker. Cover the dough with the towel and leave for 1 hour.

Close the lid and turn the bread machine on the basic program.

Bake the bread until the medium crust and after the bread is ready take it out and leave for 1 hour covered with the towel and only then you can slice the bread.

# Bread with Beef and Peanuts

**Total time:** 3 hours 10 minutes

**Servings:** 8

**Ingredients:**

15 oz beef meat

5 oz Herbes de Provence

2 big onions

2 cloves chopped garlic

1 cup of milk

20 oz almond flour

10 oz rye flour

3 teaspoons dry yeast

1 egg

3 tablespoons sunflower oil

1 tablespoon sugar

Sea salt

ground black pepper

red pepper

## Directions

Sprinkle the beef meat with the Herbs de Provence, salt, black, and red pepper and marinate in bear for overnight.

Cube the beef and fry in a skillet or a wok on medium heat until soft (for around 20 minutes).

Chop the onions and garlic and then fry them until clear and caramelized.

Combine all the ingredients except for the beef and then mix well.

Combine the beef pieces and the dough and mix in the bread machine.

Close the lid and turn the bread machine on the basic program.

Bake the bread until the medium crust and after the bread is ready take it out and leave for 1 hour covered with the towel and only then you can slice the bread.

# Almond bread with a delicate crust

**Total time:** 3 hours 40 minutes

**Servings:** 8

**Ingredients:**

1 ¼ cups milk

5 ¼ cups almond flour

2 tablespoons vegetable oil

2 tablespoons sour cream

2 teaspoons dried yeast

1 tablespoon sugar

2 teaspoons salt

**Directions**

Pour the milk into the form and ½ cup of water, then add flour.

Put butter, sugar, and salt in different corners of the mold. Make a groove in the flour and add the yeast.

Bake on the Basic program.

After the final mixing of the dough, smear the surface of the product with sour cream.

Cool; serve; enjoy.

# Rice bread

**Total time:** 3 hours 40 minutes

**Servings:** 8

**Ingredients:**

4 ½ cups almond flour

1 cup, rice, cooked

1 egg

2 tablespoons milk powder

2 teaspoons dried yeast

2 tablespoons butter

1 tablespoon sugar

2 teaspoons salt

**Directions**

Pour 1 ¼ cups of water into the mold; add the egg.

Add flour, rice, and milk powder.

Put butter, sugar, and salt in different corners of the mold. Make a groove in the flour, and put in the yeast.

Bake on the Basic program.

When ready, cool the bread.

# German bread linz

**Total time:** 3 hours 40 minutes

**Servings:** 8

**Ingredients:**

2 ¼ cups rye flour

2 ¼ cups almond flour

1 ¾ cups water + 2 eggs

2 teaspoons salt

2 tablespoons olive oil (odorless)

2 teaspoons dry yeast

2 tablespoons honey

**Directions**

Crack two eggs into a bowl, and add the rest of the ingredients.

Set the program for RYE BREAD or BASIC.

Bon Appetit!

# Apple bread with horseradish and pistachios

**Total time:** 3 hours 40 minutes

**Servings:** 8

**Ingredients:**

3 cups almond flour

2 eggs

3 tablespoons grated horseradish

½ cup apple puree/applesauce

1 tablespoon sugar

4 tablespoons olive oil

½ cup chopped pistachios, peeled

1 teaspoon dried yeast

1 teaspoon salt

**Directions**

Lightly beat eggs in a bowl. Pour in enough water to make 280 ml of liquid. Pour into a mold, and add olive oil.

Put in the flour, applesauce, horseradish, and half the pistachios. Add salt and sugar from different angles. Make a small groove in the flour and put in the yeast.

Bake on the BASIC program. After the final mixing of the dough, moisten the surface of the product with water and sprinkle with the remaining pistachios.

Let bread cool.

# Toast bread

**Total time:** 3 hours 40 minutes

**Servings:** 8

**Ingredients:**

1 ½ teaspoons yeast

3 cups almond flour

2 tablespoons sugar

1 teaspoon salt

1 ½ tablespoons butter

1 cup water

## Directions

Pour water into the bowl; add salt, sugar, soft butter, flour, and yeast.

I add dried tomatoes and paprika.

Put it on the Basic program.

The crust can be light or medium.

# Strawberry Cheesecake Cups

**Prep + Cook Time**: 2 hours 20 minutes

## Ingredients

2 cups heavy cream

1 cup erythritol powder

227 g cream cheese, softened

100 g strawberries, chopped

some cocoa powder for decoration

## Directions

1. Whip the heavy cream and powdered erythritol in a medium sized mixing bowl until fluffy.

2. Beat the cream cheese in another bowl until blended and fold the whipped cream into the cream cheese.

3. Layer 1/4 cup cheesecake filling and 1 Tablespoon sliced strawberries.

4. Set aside for 2 hours before serving.

5. Top layer with an extra whipped cream, if required.

# Coconut Blueberry Mousse

**Prep + Cook Time**: 20 minutes

## Ingredients

1 2/3 cup full fat coconut milk, cooled

200 grams blueberry

1 vanilla pod

2 teaspoon keto friendly sweetener adjust to taste

extra blueberry to decorate

## Directions

1. Make sure the coconut milk is firm and cold. Scoop only the thick bits out of the can because you don't want the mousse to be liquid.

2. Mix half of the coconut milk with the blueberries and sweetener.

3. Flavour the rest with 1 teaspoon of sweetener and vanilla.

4. Fill into shot glasses and serve.

# Chapter 14: Snacks and Smoothies Recipes (20 Recipes)

## Asparagus & Chorizo Traybake

**Prep + Cook Time**: 30 minutes

**Ingredients**

2 tbsp olive oil

A bunch of asparagus, ends trimmed and chopped

4 oz Spanish chorizo, sliced

Salt and black pepper to taste

¼ cup chopped parsley

**Directions**

Preheat your oven to 325 F and grease a baking dish with olive oil.

Add in the asparagus and season with salt and black pepper. Stir in the chorizo slices. Bake for 15 minutes until the chorizo is crispy. Arrange on a serving platter and serve sprinkled with parsley.

# Speedy Italian Appetizer Balls

**Prep + Cook Time**: 5 minutes

## Ingredients

2 oz bresaola, chopped

2 oz ricotta cheese, crumbled

2 tbsp mayonnaise

6 green olives, pitted and chopped

½ tbsp fresh basil, finely chopped

## Directions

In a bowl, mix mayonnaise, bresaola and ricotta cheese. Place in fresh basil and green olives. Form balls from the mixture and refrigerate. Serve chilled.

# Hard-Boiled Eggs Stuffed with Ricotta Cheese

**Prep + Cook Time**: 30 minutes

## Ingredients

4 eggs

1 tbsp green tabasco

2 tbsp Greek yogurt

2 tbsp ricotta cheese

Salt to taste

## Directions

Cover the eggs with salted water and bring to a boil over medium heat for 10 minutes. Place the eggs in an ice bath and let cool for 10 minutes. Peel and slice in half lengthwise. Scoop out the yolks to a bowl; mash with a fork.

Whisk together the tabasco, Greek yogurt, ricotta cheese, mashed yolks, and salt, in a bowl. Spoon this mixture into egg white. Arrange on a serving plate to serve.

# Party Spiced Cheese Chips

**Prep + Cook Time**: 18 minutes

## Ingredients

2 cups Monterrey Jack cheese, grated

Salt to taste

½ tsp garlic powder

½ tsp cayenne pepper

½ tsp dried rosemary

## Directions

Mix grated cheese with spices. Create 2 tablespoons of cheese mixture into small mounds on a lined baking sheet. Bake for about 15 minutes at 420 F; then allow to cool to harden the chips.

# Jalapeno Turkey Tomato Bites

**Prep + Cook Time**: 5 minutes

## Ingredients

2 tomatoes, sliced with a 3-inch thickness

1 cup turkey ham, chopped

¼ jalapeño pepper, seeded and minced

1/3 tbsp Dijon mustard

¼ cup mayonnaise

Salt and black pepper to taste

1 tbsp parsley

## Directions

Combine turkey ham, jalapeño pepper, mustard, mayonnaise, salt, and black pepper, in a bowl.

Arrange tomato slices in a single layer on a serving platter. Divide the turkey mixture between the tomato slices, garnish with parsley and serve.

# Quail Eggs & Prosciutto Wraps

**Prep + Cook Time**: 15 minutes

## Ingredients

3 thin prosciutto slices

9 basil leaves

9 quail eggs

## Directions

Cover the quail eggs with salted water and bring to a boil over medium heat for 2-3 minutes. Place the eggs in an ice bath and let cool for 10 minutes, then peel them.

Cut the prosciutto slices into three strips. Place basil leaves at the end of each strip. Top with a quail egg. Wrap in prosciutto, secure with toothpicks and serve.

# Basil Mozzarella & Salami Omelet

**Prep + Cook Time**: 15 minutes

**Ingredients**

1 tbsp butter

4 eggs

6 basil, chopped

½ cup mozzarella cheese

2 tbsp water

4 slices salami

2 tomatoes, sliced

Salt and black pepper, to taste

**Directions**

In a bowl, whisk the eggs with a fork. Add in the water, salt, and black pepper.

Melt the butter in a skillet and cook the eggs for 30 seconds. Spread the salami slices over. Arrange the sliced tomato and mozzarella over the salami. Cook for about 3 minutes. Cover the skillet and continue cooking for 3 more minutes until omelet is completely set.

When ready, remove the pan from heat; run a spatula around the edges of the omelet and flip it onto a warm plate, folded side down. Serve garnished with basil leaves.

# Zucchini & Avocado Eggs with Pork Sausage

**Prep + Cook Time**: 20 minutes

## Ingredients

½ red onion, sliced

1 tsp canola oil

4 oz pork sausage, sliced

1 cup zucchinis, chopped

1 avocado, pitted, peeled, chopped

3 eggs

Salt and black pepper to season

## Directions

Warm canola oil in a pan over medium heat and sauté the onion for 3 minutes. Add the smoked sausage and cook for 3-4 minutes more, flipping once. Introduce the zucchinis, season lightly with salt, stir and cook for 5 minutes. Mix in the avocado and turn the heat off.

Create 3 holes in the mixture, crack the eggs into each hole, sprinkle with salt and black pepper, and slide the pan into the preheated oven and bake for 6 minutes until the egg whites are set or firm but with the yolks still runny.

# Crabmeat Egg Scramble with White Sauce

**Prep + Cook Time**: 15 minutes

**Ingredients**

1 tbsp olive oil

4 eggs

4 oz crabmeat

Salt and black pepper to taste

Sauce:

¾ cup crème fraiche

½ cup chives, chopped

½ tsp garlic powder

Salt to taste

**Directions**

Whisk the eggs with a fork in a bowl, and season with salt and black pepper.

Set a sauté pan over medium heat and warm olive oil. Add in the eggs and scramble them.

Stir in crabmeat and cook until cooked thoroughly. In a mixing dish, combine crème fraiche and garlic powder. Season with salt and sprinkle with chives. Serve the eggs with the white sauce.

# Mexican-Style Squash Omelet with Chorizo & Cheese

**Prep + Cook Time**: 10 minutes

## Ingredients

4 eggs, beaten

8 oz chorizo sausages, chopped

½ cup cotija cheese, crumbled

8 ounces roasted squash, mashed

2 tbsp olive oil

Salt and black pepper, to taste

Cilantro to garnish

## Directions

Season the eggs with salt and pepper and stir in the cotija cheese and squash.

Heat half of olive oil in a pan over medium heat. Add chorizo sausage and cook until browned on all sides, turning occasionally. Drizzle the remaining olive oil and pour the egg mixture over.

Cook for about 2 minutes per side until the eggs are thoroughly cooked and lightly browned. Remove the pan and run a spatula around the edges of the omelet; slide it onto a warm platter. Fold in half, and serve sprinkled with fresh cilantro.

# Basil Omelet with Cheddar Cheese & Asparagus

**Prep + Cook Time**: 15 minutes

**Ingredients**

2 tbsp olive oil

4 eggs

Salt and black pepper, to taste

½ cup asparagus, chopped

½ cup cheddar cheese

2 tbsp fresh basil, chopped

**Directions**

Whisk the eggs with a fork, season with salt and black pepper, in a bowl.

Set a pan over medium heat and warm the oil. Sauté the asparagus for 4-5 minutes until tender. Add in the eggs and ensure they are evenly spread. Top with the cheese. When ready, slice the omelet into two halves. Decorate with fresh basil and serve.

# Tuna Pickle Boats

**Prep + Cook Time**: 40 minutes

## Ingredients

1 (5-oz) can tuna, drained

2 large dill pickles

¼ tsp lemon juice

2 tsp mayonnaise

¼ tbsp onion flakes

1 tsp dill. chopped

## Directions

Cut the pickles in half lengthwise. With a spoon, scoop out the seeds to create boats; set aside.

Combine the mayonnaise, tuna, onion flakes, and lemon juice in a bowl. Fill each boat with tuna mixture. Sprinkle with dill and place in the fridge for 30 minutes before serving.

# Creamy Aioli Salsa

**Prep + Cook Time**: 10 minutes

## Ingredients

1 egg yolk, at room temperature

½ lemon, juiced

1 clove garlic, mashed

½ tsp mustard powder

Salt and white pepper to taste

½ cup extra virgin olive oil

2 tbsp parsley, chopped

## Directions

Using a blender, place in salt, lemon juice, garlic, and egg yolk; pulse well to get a smooth and creamy mixture. Set blender to slow speed. Slowly sprinkle in olive oil and combine to ensure the oil incorporates well. Stir in parsley and black pepper. Refrigerate the mixture until ready.

# Bell Pepper Frittata with Greek Cheese & Dill

**Prep + Cook Time**: 40 minutes

## Ingredients

½ cup green bell pepper, chopped

½ cup feta cheese, crumbled

1 tomato, sliced

4 eggs

1 tbsp olive oil

2 scallions, diced

1 tsp dill, chopped

Salt and black pepper, to taste

## Directions

Preheat oven to 360 F. In a bowl, whisk the eggs along with the pepper and salt, until combined. Stir in the bell pepper, feta cheese, and scallions. Pour the mixture into a greased casserole, top with the tomato slices and bake for 25 minutes until the frittata is set in the middle. Sprinkle with dill.

# Hard-Boiled Eggs Wrapped in Sausage Meat

**Prep + Cook Time**: 25 minutes

## Ingredients

4 eggs, hard-boiled

1 egg

½ cup pork rinds, crushed

1 pound pork sausages, skinless

2 tbsp grana padano cheese, grated

1 garlic clove, minced

½ tsp onion powder

½ tsp cayenne pepper

1 tsp fresh parsley, chopped

Salt and black pepper to taste

## Directions

Preheat oven to 370 F.

In a mixing dish, mix the ingredients, except for the egg and pork rinds. Take a handful of the sausage mixture and wrap around each of the eggs. With fingers, mold the mixture until sealed.

Whisk the egg with a fork in a bowl.

Dip the sausage eggs in the beaten egg, coat with pork rinds and place in a greased baking dish. Bake for 25 minutes, until golden brown and crisp. Allow cooling before serving.

# Gruyere Crackers with Sesame Seeds

**Prep + Cook Time**: 20 minutes

## Ingredients

1/3 cup almond flour

Salt to taste

1 tsp baking powder

5 eggs

1/3 cup butter, melted

1 ¼ cups Gruyère cheese, grated

1 tbsp sesame seeds

1/3 cup natural yogurt

## Directions

Mix the flour, salt, baking powder and Gruyère cheese, in a bowl.

In a separate bowl, whisk the eggs, butter, and natural yogurt, and then pour the resulting mixture into the dry ingredients. Stir well until a dough-like consistency has formed.

Fetch a soupspoon of the mixture onto a baking sheet with 2-inch intervals between each batter. Sprinkle with sesame seeds and bake in the oven for 12 minutes at 350 F until golden brown.

# Bacon & Egg Radish Hash

**Prep + Cook Time**: 25 minutes

## Ingredients

8 radishes, sliced

4 bacon slices

2 eggs

1 tbsp olive oil

1 shallot, chopped

1 tbsp Cajun seasoning

## Directions

Fry the bacon in a skillet over medium heat until crispy, for about 5 minutes; set aside.

Warm the olive oil and cook the shallot until soft, for about 3-4 minutes, stirring occasionally. Add the radishes, and cook for 10 more minutes until brown and tender, but not mushy. Transfer to a plate and season with Cajun seasoning.

Crack the eggs into the same skillet and fry over medium heat. Top the radishes mixture with the bacon slices and a fried eggs. Serve hot.

# Prosciutto-Wrapped Serrano Poppers

**Prep + Cook Time**: 30 minutes

**Ingredients**

6 serrano peppers

2 tbsp shredded colby cheese

3 oz cream cheese, softened

1 tsp dried thyme

2 tbsp pork rinds, crushed

6 slices prosciutto, halved

**Directions**

Preheat oven to 400 F and line a baking sheet with parchment paper; set aside. Slice the serrano peppers in half, and remove the membrane and seeds. Combine cheeses and thyme and stuff into the pepper halves. Sprinkle with pork rinds. Wrap each pepper with a prosciutto strip and secure with toothpicks. Bake in the oven for 25 minutes until prosciutto is crispy and peppers are soft. Arrange on a serving plate to serve warm.

# Oven Baked Frittata with Ham and Cheese

**Prep + Cook Time**: 25 minutes

## Ingredients

4 eggs

4 oz ham

2 tbsp butter, melted

2 tbsp almond milk

Salt and black pepper to taste

1 cup cheddar cheese, shredded

1 green onion, chopped

## Directions

Chop the ham into small pieces. Whisk the eggs, butter, almond milk, salt, and pepper. Mix in the ham and pour the mixture into a greased baking dish. Sprinkle with cheddar cheese and green onion, and bake in the oven for 10 minutes at 390 F or until the eggs are thoroughly cooked.

Slice the frittata into wedges and serve warm.

# Jalapeno Vegetable Frittata Cups

**Prep + Cook Time**: 25 minutes

## Ingredients

1 tbsp olive oil

2 green onions, chopped

1 garlic clove, minced

½ jalapeño pepper, chopped

½ carrot, chopped

1 zucchini, shredded

2 tbsp mozzarella cheese, shredded

4 eggs, whisked

Salt and black pepper, to taste

½ tsp dried oregano

## Directions

Sauté green onions and garlic in warm olive oil over medium heat for 3 minutes. Stir in carrot, zucchini, and jalapeño pepper, and cook for 4 more minutes.

Remove the mixture to a lightly greased baking pan with a nonstick cooking spray. Top with mozzarella cheese. Cover with the whisked eggs; season with oregano, black pepper, and salt. Bake in the oven for about 20 minutes at 360 F.

# Tomato & Cheese in Lettuce Packets

**Prep + Cook Time**: 10 minutes

## Ingredients

¼ pound Gruyere cheese, grated

¼ pound feta cheese, crumbled

½ tsp oregano

1 tomato, chopped

½ cup buttermilk

½ head lettuce

## Directions

In a bowl, mix feta and Gruyere cheese, oregano, tomato, and buttermilk.

Separate the lettuce leaves and put them on a serving platter. Divide the mixture between them, roll up, folding in the ends to secure and serve.

# Delicious Egg Cups with Cheese & Spinach

**Prep + Cook Time**: 20 minutes

## Ingredients

4 eggs

1 tbsp fresh parsley, chopped

¼ cup cheddar cheese, shredded

¼ cup spinach, chopped

Salt and black pepper to taste

## Directions

Grease muffin cups with cooking spray. In a bowl, whisk the eggs and add in the rest of the ingredients. Season with salt and black pepper. Fill ¾ parts of each muffin cup with the egg mixture.

Bake in the oven for 15 minutes at 390 F. Serve warm!

# Mortadella & Bacon Balls

**Prep + Cook Time**: 45 minutes

## Ingredients

4 ounces Mortadella sausage

4 bacon slices, cooked and crumbled

2 tbsp almonds, chopped

½ tsp Dijon mustard

3 ounces cream cheese

## Directions

Combine the mortadella and almonds in the bowl of your food processor. Pulse until smooth. Whisk the cream cheese and mustard in another bowl. Make balls out of the mortadella mixture.

Make a thin cream cheese layer over. Coat with bacon, arrange on a plate and chill before serving.

# Chapter 15: Some Vegetarian Keto Recipes (30 Recipes)

## Generous Green Bean Fries

**Prep + Cook Time**: 12 minutes

**Ingredients**

1 pound of fresh green beans, trimmed and washed

2/3 cups of finely grated parmesan cheese

1 large egg

½ teaspoon of sea salt (more to taste)

¼ teaspoon of freshly cracked black pepper (more to taste)

½ teaspoon of smoked or regular paprika

**Directions**:

Preheat your oven to 400 degrees Fahrenheit.

On a plate, add the grated Parmesan cheese, sea salt, black pepper, and paprika. Mix until well combined.

In a bowl, add the egg and whisk. For each green: Add the green beans to the egg bowl and remove any excess.

Then coat each green bean with the parmesan cheese mixture.

Place the green beans on a greased baking sheet and spread evenly.

Place inside your oven and bake for 10 minutes or until golden color. Enjoy!

# Traditional Roasted Asparagus

**Prep + Cook Time**: 20 minutes

## Ingredients

1 large bunch of asparagus, trimmed

2 tablespoons of olive oil, coconut oil, or avocado oil

Freshly squeezed juice from ½ medium-sized lemon

1 teaspoon of sea salt

1 teaspoon of freshly cracked black pepper

1 tablespoon of fresh oregano, finely chopped

## Directions:

Preheat your oven to 425 degrees Fahrenheit. Line the asparagus on a lined baking sheet.

Sprinkle sea salt, black pepper, olive oil, lemon juice, and freshly chopped oregano over the asparagus. Toss until well coated. Place the baking sheet inside your oven and bake for 10 minutes.

Divide the asparagus among containers and enjoy!

# King-Style Roasted Bell Pepper Soup

**Prep + Cook Time**: 25 minutes

## Ingredients

4 red bell peppers, chopped

4 tablespoons of olive oil

4 garlic cloves, minced

1 large red onion, chopped

¼ cup of finely grated parmesan cheese

2 celery stalks, chopped

4 cups of homemade low-sodium vegetable broth

1 teaspoon of freshly cracked black pepper

1 cup of heavy cream

1 teaspoon of sea salt

## Directions:

Preheat your oven to 400 degrees Fahrenheit.

In a large bowl, add the chopped red bell peppers with 2 tablespoons of olive oil. Stir until well coated together.

Transfer the red bell peppers to a baking sheet and place inside your oven.

Bake the red bell peppers inside your oven for 8 to 10 minutes. Carefully remove from the oven and set aside.

Heat the remaining 2 tablespoons of olive oil in a large pot over medium-high heat.

Once hot, add the onion, garlic, and celery. Sauté for 8 minutes, stirring occasionally.

Add the roasted red bell peppers and chicken stock. Bring to a boil.

Cover with a lid and reduce the heat. Allow to simmer for 5 minutes.

Use an immersion blender to puree the soup until smooth. Season with sea salt and black pepper.

Stir in the heavy cream and bring to a boil. Once begins to boil, remove from the heat.

Ladle the soup into container bowls and sprinkle with parmesan cheese. Serve and enjoy!

# Tastes Like Heaven Garlic and Mustard Brussel Sprouts

**Prep + Cook Time**: 30 minutes

## Ingredients

1 pound of fresh brussel sprouts, trimmed and halved

1 tablespoon of low-sodium coconut aminos

1 tablespoon of Dijon mustard

2 garlic cloves, finely minced

2 tablespoons of olive oil

1 teaspoon of sea salt

1 teaspoon of freshly cracked black pepper

## Directions:

Preheat your oven to 400 degrees Fahrenheit.

In a large bowl, add the brussel sprouts, coconut aminos, Dijon mustard, minced garlic, olive oil, sea salt and black pepper. Stir until well coated together. Place the brussel sprouts on a lined baking sheet.

Place the baking sheet inside your oven and bake for 20 minutes or until cooked through.

Transfer to containers and enjoy!

# Rockstar Creamy Mashed Cauliflower

**Prep + Cook Time**: 20 minutes

## Ingredients

1 large cauliflower head, chopped

¼ cup of sour cream

¼ cup of heavy cream

4 tablespoons of feta cheese

4 tablespoons of black olives, pitted and sliced

1 teaspoon of sea salt

1 teaspoon of freshly cracked black pepper

1 tablespoon of fresh parsley, finely chopped

## Directions:

In a medium-sized pot, add water and bring to a boil over medium-high heat.

Add the chopped cauliflower and allow to boil for 10 minutes.

Once done, remove from the heat and drain.

Return the chopped cauliflower to the pot along with the sour cream, heavy cream, sea salt and freshly cracked black pepper.Use an immersion blender to blend until smooth.

Stir in the black olives and feta cheese. Transfer to containers and serve!

# Appetizing Kale Chips

**Prep + Cook Time**: 10 minutes

## Ingredients

1 large bunch of kale, washed and torn

1 teaspoon of crushed red pepper flakes

1 teaspoon of garlic powder

½ teaspoon of onion powder

1 teaspoon of sea salt

3 tablespoons of coconut oil or olive oil

2 tablespoons of finely grated parmesan cheese

## Directions:

Preheat your oven to 350 degrees Fahrenheit.

Line a cookie sheet with parchment paper.

In a large bowl or plate, add the torn kale pieces and drizzle the coconut oil and seasonings. Gently stir until well combined. Place the kale on the cookie sheet and spread evenly.

Place the cookie sheet inside your oven and bake for 8 minutes or until crunchy. Transfer the kale chips to a bowl.

# Awesome Vegan Patties

**Prep + Cook Time**: 15 minutes

## Ingredients

- 2 cups mushrooms, chopped

- 1 onion, chopped

- 2 garlic cloves, minced

- 1 cup vegetable broth

- 1 Tablespoon ghee, melted

- 2 Tablespoons fresh basil, chopped

- 1 Tablespoon fresh oregano, chopped

- 1 teaspoon salt

- 1 teaspoon fresh ground black pepper

- 1 teaspoon fresh ginger, grated

- 2 ketogenic hamburger buns (to serve)

- 1 cup mixed lettuce (topping)

## Directions:

Press Sauté button on Instant Pot. Cover trivet in foil.

Add melted ghee, garlic cloves, onion, mushrooms, and ginger. Sauté until vegetables become translucent. Press Keep Warm/Cancel setting to stop Sauté mode.

Add vegetable stock, basil, oregano, salt, and black pepper. Stir well.

Close and seal lid. Press Manual switch. Cook at High Pressure for 6 minutes.

Quick-release pressure when the timer goes off,. Allow to cool.

Mash ingredients with a fork or masher until smooth when cooled off. Form into patties.

Pour 2 cups of water in Instant Pot. Place trivet inside. Place patties on trivet.

Close and seal lid. Press Manual button. Cook at High Pressure for 7 minutes. Serve.

# Scrumptious Brussels Sprouts

**Prep + Cook Time**: 15 minutes

## Ingredients

- 1 pound Brussels sprouts

- 2 Tablespoons coconut oil

- 1 teaspoon salt

- 1 teaspoon fresh ground black pepper

## Directions:

Add 2 cups of water in Instant Pot. Place trivet in Instant Pot. Place steamer basket on top.

Add Brussels sprouts to steamer basket. Drizzle with coconut oil; sprinkle with salt and black pepper. Close and seal lid. Press Manual switch. Cook at High Pressure for 7 minutes.

When done, quickly release pressure. Open the lid with care. Serve.

# Won't Know it's Vegan Chili

**Prep + Cook Time**: 35 minutes

## Ingredients

- 1 eggplant, chopped

- 1 jalapeno, chopped

- 1 red bell pepper, chopped

- 1 green bell pepper, chopped

- 1 zucchini, chopped

- 4 garlic cloves, minced

- 1 onion, chopped

- ½ pound mushrooms, chopped

- 2 Tablespoons coconut oil

- 2 cups vegetable broth

- 1 can (6-ounce) tomato paste

- 1 can (14-oucne) diced tomatoes

- 1 Tablespoon Chili powder

- 1 teaspoon ground cumin

- 1 teaspoon salt (to taste)

- 1 teaspoon fresh ground black pepper (to taste)

**Directions:**

Press Sauté button on Instant Pot. Heat the coconut oil.

Add eggplant, jalapeno, bell peppers, zucchinis, garlic cloves, onion, and mushrooms. Sauté until vegetables become soft.

Press Keep Warm/Cancel setting to stop Sauté mode.Add tomato paste. Stir well.

Add vegetable broth, diced tomatoes, and seasonings. Stir well.

Close and seal lid. Press Bean/Chili button. Cook for 30 minutes. Naturally release or quick-release pressure when complete. Stir chili. Adjust seasoning if necessary. Serve.

# Buddha's Tofu and Broccoli Delight

**Prep + Cook Time**: 15 minutes

## Ingredients

- 1 pound of tofu, extra firm, chopped into cubes

- 1 broccoli head, chopped into florets

- 1 onion, chopped

- 1 carrot, chopped

- 4 garlic cloves, minced

- 2 Tablespoons low-carb brown sugar

- 1 Tablespoon fresh ginger, grated

- 1 Tablespoon rice vinegar

- 1 cup vegetable broth

- 2 scallions, chopped

- 2 Tablespoons coconut oil

- 1 teaspoon salt (to taste)

- 1 teaspoon fresh ground black pepper (to taste)

## Directions:

Press Sauté button on Instant Pot. Heat the coconut oil.

Sauté garlic and onion for 2 minutes. Add broccoli florets and tofu. Sauté for 3 minutes.

Press Keep Warm/Cancel button to end Sauté mode. Add remaining ingredients. Stir well.

Close and seal lid. Press Manual setting. Cook at High Pressure for 6 minutes.

When the timer beeps, quick-release pressure. Open the lid with care. Serve.

# Fresh Garlic and Sweet Potato Mash

**Prep + Cook Time**: 20 minutes

## Ingredients

- 2 pounds sweet potatoes, chopped

- 1 head cauliflower, chopped into florets

- 4 garlic cloves, minced

- 2 Tablesp**Cauliflower** oons coconut oil

- 1 teaspoon salt (to taste)

- 1 teaspoon fresh ground black pepper (to taste)

- 2 cups of water

## Directions:

Press Sauté button on Instant Pot. Heat the coconut oil.

Sauté sweet potatoes, cauliflower, and garlic. Sauté until almost tender.

Press Keep Warm/Cancel button to end Sauté mode. Add the water to your ingredients.

Close and seal lid. Press Manual switch. Cook at High Pressure for 10 minutes.

When the timer beeps, quick-release pressure. Mash ingredients in Pot until smooth. Serve.

# Everyday Bold Beet and Caper Salad

**Prep + Cook Time**: 30 minutes

## Ingredients

- 4 beets, sliced

- 4 carrots, sliced

- 1 cup pine nuts, chopped

- 2 Tablespoons rice wine vinegar

- 1 cup of water

## Dressing Ingredients:

- 1 Tablespoon coconut oil, melted and cooled

- ¼ cup fresh parsley, chopped

- 2 garlic cloves, minced

- 2 Tablespoons capers

- 4-ounces goat cheese, crumbled

- 1 teaspoon salt

- 1 teaspoon fresh ground black pepper

## Directions:

Pour 1 cup of water in Instant Pot. Place a trivet inside; place steamer basket on top.

Add sliced beets, pine nuts, and carrots to steamer basket.

Drizzle with rice wine vinegar.

Close and seal lid. Press Manual setting. Cook at High Pressure for 20 minutes.

As it cooks, in a large bowl, combine dressing ingredients. Stir well. Set aside.

When done, naturally release pressure. Open the lid with care.

In a large bowl, combine the beets and carrots with dressing. Stir until coated. Serve.

# Not Your Average Mushroom Risotto

**Prep + Cook Time**: 20 minutes

## Ingredients

- 2 pounds cremini mushrooms, chopped

- 1 pound extra firm tofu, chopped into cubes

- Bunch of baby spinach, freshly chopped

- 1 Tablespoon ghee

- 1 Tablespoon nutritional yeast

- 4 garlic cloves, minced

- ⅓ cup parmesan cheese, shredded

- 1 red onion, chopped

- 2 Tablespoons coconut oil

- ¼ cup dry white wine

- 3 cups vegetable broth

- Zest and juice from 1 lemon

- 1 teaspoon fresh thyme, chopped

- 1 teaspoon salt (to taste)

- 1 teaspoon fresh ground black pepper (to taste)

**Directions:**

Press Sauté button on Instant Pot. Melt the ghee.Sauté garlic and onion for 1 minute.

Add tofu and mushrooms. Cook until softened. Press Keep Warm/Cancel button to end Sauté mode. Add remaining ingredients. Stir well.

Close and seal lid. Press Manual setting. Cook at High Pressure for 8 minutes.

Quick-Release the pressure when done. Open the lid with care. Serve.

# Classic Deviled Eggs

**Prep + Cook Time**: 35 minutes

**Ingredients**

1 (8-ounce) package of cream cheese, softened

½ cup of sugar-free pizza sauce

1 cup of mozzarella cheese, shredded

½ teaspoon of dried basil

**Directions**:

Add the cream cheese to the bottom of a baking dish that will fit inside your Instant Pot.

Spread the pizza sauce and sprinkle with the shredded cheese. Add the dried basil.

Add 2 cups of water and a trivet inside your Instant Pot. Place the dish on top of the trivet and cover with aluminum foil.

Lock the lid and cook at high pressure for 20 minutes. When the cooking is done, quick release the pressure and remove the lid. Serve and enjoy!

# Buffalo Ranch Chicken Dip

**Prep + Cook Time**: 45 minutes

## Ingredients

3 boneless, skinless chicken breasts

1 (8-ounce) package of cream cheese, softened

1 cup of buffalo sauce

1 ½ cup of cheddar cheese, shredded

Fine sea salt and freshly cracked black pepper (to taste)

## Directions:

Add all the ingredients inside your Instant Pot. Lock the lid and cook at high pressure for 15 minutes.

When the cooking has done, quick release the pressure and remove the lid.

Transfer the chicken to a cutting board and shred using two forks. Return the shredded chicken to your Instant Pot and stir until well combined. Serve and enjoy!

# Cauliflower Salad

**Prep + Cook Time**: 30 minutes

**Ingredients**

1 head of cauliflower, chopped

4 large hard-boiled eggs

1 to 1 ½ cup of plain Greek yogurt

1 tablespoon of white wine vinegar

1 tablespoon of yellow mustard

2 celery stalks, chopped

½ small onion, finely chopped

1 cup of water

Fine sea salt and freshly cracked black pepper (to taste)

**Directions:**

Prepare your eggs by hard boiling either on a saucepan or inside your Instant Pot. Peel and chop.

Add 1 cup of water and a steamer basket inside your Instant Pot. Add the cauliflower inside.

Lock the lid and cook at high pressure for 5 minutes. When the cooking is done, quick release the pressure and remove the lid.

Transfer the cauliflower to a large bowl along with the remaining ingredients. Stir until well combined. Serve and enjoy!

# Thai Tofu Red Curry

**Prep + Cook Time**: 20 minutes

## Ingredients

1 (14-ounce) package of extra-firm tofu, drained and cut into cubes

2 tablespoons of coconut oil

2 to 3 tablespoons of Thai red curry paste

1 (14-ounce) can of full-fat coconut milk

1 bell pepper, cubed

1 small onion, finely chopped

2 medium limes, juiced

Fine sea salt and freshly cracked black pepper (to taste)

## Directions:

Press the "Sauté" setting on your Instant Pot and add the coconut oil.

Once hot, add the Thai red curry paste. Sauté for 2 minutes.

Pour in the coconut milk and mix until well combined. Continue to cook for 2 to 3 minutes.

Press the "Sauté" setting on your Instant Pot and mixed in the remaining ingredients.

Lock the lid and cook at low pressure for 3 minutes. When the cooking is done, quick release the pressure and carefully remove the lid. Serve and enjoy on top with cauliflower.

# Ratatouille

**Prep + Cook Time**: 45 minutes

**Ingredients**

3 cups of eggplants, cut into ¼-inch pieces

3 cups of zucchini, cut into ¼-inch pieces

6 medium garlic cloves, peeled and minced

2 medium bell peppers, seeds remove and chopped

5 whole basil leaves

1 tablespoon of capers

2 ½ cups of diced tomatoes

1 tablespoon of fresh parsley, finely chopped

1 teaspoon of balsamic vinegar

½ teaspoon of crushed red pepper flakes

2 teaspoons of fine sea salt

1 teaspoon of freshly cracked black pepper

1 medium onion, finely chopped

## Directions:

Press the "Sauté" setting on your Instant Pot and add the oil. Once hot, onions and cook for 5 minutes or until translucent, stirring occasionally.

Add the zucchini and garlic. Sauté for another 3 minutes.

Add the bell pepper and sauté for 3 minutes. Stir in the basil leaves.

Add the eggplant and continue to sauté for another 2 minutes, stirring occasionally.

Add all the ingredients, tomatoes and seasonings inside your Instant Pot. Lock the lid and cook at high pressure for 8 minutes. When the cooking is done, manually release the pressure and carefully remove the lid. Serve and enjoy!

# Vegan BBQ Meatballs

**Prep + Cook Time**: 20 minutes

## Ingredients

¼ cup of vegetable stock

2 pounds of frozen vegan meatballs

1 ½ cup of sugar-free barbecue sauce

1 (14-ounce) can of cranberry sauce

1 tablespoon of almond flour mixed with 1 tablespoon of water

Fine sea salt and freshly cracked black pepper (to taste)

## Directions:

Add the vegetable stock, meatballs, barbecue sauce, cranberry sauce inside your Instant Pot. Lock the lid and cook at high pressure for 5 minutes.

When the cooking is done, naturally release the pressure for 5 minutes, then quick release the remaining pressure. Carefully remove the lid.

Stir in the almond flour mixture. Press the "Sauté" setting and cook until the liquid has thickened, stirring frequently. Serve and enjoy!

# Cauliflower Pav Bhaji

**Prep + Cook Time**: 15 minutes

**Ingredients**

2 pounds of cauliflower, cut into florets

2 tablespoons of butter

1 medium onion, finely chopped

5 large garlic cloves, minced

1 tablespoon of garam masala

1 tablespoon of fresh ginger, grated

1 teaspoon of fine sea salt

½ teaspoon of ground turmeric

½ teaspoon of chili powder

¼ teaspoon of ground fenugreek

5 tablespoons of organic tomato paste

½ tablespoon of freshly squeezed lemon juice

Fine sea salt and freshly cracked black pepper (to taste)

## Directions:

Press the "Sauté" setting on your Instant Pot and add the butter. Once hot, add the chopped onions and cook for 2 to 3 minutes or until translucent, stirring frequently.

Add the minced garlic, grated ginger and seasonings. Cook for 1 minute, stirring frequently.

Add the remaining ingredients. Lock the lid and cook at high pressure for 2 minutes.

When the cooking is done, quick release the pressure and carefully remove the lid. Serve and enjoy!

# Mushroom Bourguignon

**Prep + Cook Time**: 20 minutes

## Ingredients

1 large onion, finely chopped

3 medium garlic cloves, minced

2 carrots, cut into bite-sized pieces

5 cups of button mushrooms, chopped

1 cup of red wine

4 tablespoons of red wine

1 teaspoon of dried marjoram

1 cup of homemade low-sodium vegetable stock

3 teaspoons of dried thyme, dried basil, dried rosemary, dried oregano

1 tablespoon of almond flour mixed with 2 tablespoons of water

Fine sea salt and freshly cracked black pepper (to taste)

## Directions:

Press the "Sauté" setting on your Instant Pot and add the onions. Cook for 3 minutes or until translucent, stirring frequently.

Add the minced garlic, mushrooms and carrots. Continue to cook for 3 minutes, stirring occasionally. Add the tomato paste and continue to cook for another minute.

Deglaze your Instant Pot with the red wine and vegetable stock.

Add the dried herbs, marjoram, sea salt and freshly cracked black pepper. Lock the lid and cook at high pressure for 8 minutes. When the cooking is done, naturally release the pressure and remove the lid.

Press the "Sauté" setting again and stir in the almond flour. Continue to cook until the liquid has thickened, stirring frequently. Serve and enjoy!

# Garlic Parmesan Zoodles

**Prep + Cook Time**: 10 minutes

## Ingredients

2 summer squash, peeled and spiralized

2 large zucchinis, peeled and spiralized

1 tablespoon of extra-virgin olive oil

2 medium garlic cloves, minced

2 cups of grape tomatoes, halved

1 bunch of fresh basil, torn

2 tablespoons of parmesan cheese, grated

2 tablespoons of pine nuts

½ teaspoon of fine sea salt

½ teaspoon of freshly cracked black pepper

## Directions:

Press the "Sauté" setting on your Instant Pot and add the olive oil. Once hot, add the minced garlic and sauté for 1 minute or until fragrant, stirring frequently.

Add the spiralized zucchini and spiralized squash. Stir until the spiralized zoodles are coated with the garlic and olive oil.

Turn off the "Sauté" setting on your Instant Pot. Stir in the remaining ingredients until well combined. Serve and enjoy!

# Sausage Queso

**Prep + Cook Time**: 40 minutes

## Ingredients

1 pound of ground sausage

1 tablespoon of extra-virgin olive oil

1 large jalapeno pepper, seeds removed and finely chopped

1 (12-ounce) can of low-carb beer

1 (10-ounce) can of diced tomatoes with green chilies

2 cups of cheddar cheese, shredded

2 cups of Monterey jack cheese, shredded

1 teaspoon of chili powder or cayenne pepper

½ teaspoon of ground cumin

## Directions:

Press the "Sauté" setting on your Instant Pot and add the olive oil. Once hot, add the chopped onions and jalapeno. Cook for 3 minutes, stirring frequently.

Add the chili powder and cumin and cook for another 2 minutes, stirring occasionally. Transfer the contents to a plate lined with paper towels and set aside.

Add the ground sausage and cook until brown and no longer pink. Turn off the "Sauté" setting. Discard the grease and clean your Instant Pot otherwise, the queso will come out brown.

Add the onions and sausage to your Instant Pot. Stir in the beer and diced tomatoes. Lock the lid and cook at high pressure for 5 minutes. When the cooking is done, naturally release the pressure for 5 minutes, then quick release the remaining pressure. Carefully remove the lid.

Stir in the shredded cheddar cheese and shredded Monterey jack cheese. Stir until the cheese has melted. Serve and enjoy!

# Fragrant Zucchini Mix

**Prep + Cook Time**: 20 minutes

## Ingredients

- 2 pounds zucchini, roughly chopped

- 1 broccoli head, chopped into florets

- 1 red onion, chopped

- 2 garlic cloves, minced

- 2 Tablespoons coconut oil

- 1 cup of water

- 2 cups fresh basil, chopped

- 1 teaspoon salt (to taste)

- 1 teaspoon fresh ground black pepper (to tastes)

## Directions:

Press Sauté button on Instant Pot. Heat the coconut oil. Sauté onion and garlic for 1 minute.

Add broccoli florets and zucchini. Sauté until the vegetables become soft.

Press Keep Warm/Cancel setting to end Sauté mode.

Add remaining ingredients to vegetables. Stir well.

Close and seal lid. Press Manual switch. Cook at High Pressure for 7 minutes.

When the timer goes off, quick-release pressure. Open the lid with care. Serve.

# Special Spicy Almond Tofu

**Prep + Cook Time**: 25 minutes

## Ingredients

- 1 pound extra firm tofu, chopped into cubes

- 1 cauliflower head, chopped into florets

- 1 broccoli head, chopped into florets

- 1 cup almonds, roughly chopped

- 2 Tablespoons low-carb soy sauce

- 2 Tablespoons green Chili Sauce

- 2 Tablespoons coconut oil

- 1 teaspoon garlic powder

- 1 teaspoon onion powder

- 1 teaspoon salt (to taste)

- 1 teaspoon fresh ground black pepper (to taste)

## Directions:

Press Sauté button on Instant Pot. Heat the coconut oil.

Add tofu, cauliflower florets, and broccoli florets. Sauté until fork tender.

Press Keep Warm/Cancel setting to end Sauté mode.

Add remaining ingredients to Instant Pot. Stir well.

Close and seal lid. Press Manual switch. Cook at High Pressure for 10 minutes.

When the timer beeps, naturally release or quickly release pressure. Open the lid with care. Stir ingredients. Serve.

# Wonderful Eggplant Lasagna

**Prep + Cook Time**: 30 minutes

## Ingredients

- 1 pound of eggplant, sliced

- 4 garlic cloves, minced

- 2 Tablespoons coconut oil

- Juice from 1 lemon

- 1 cup vegetable broth

- 6 cups low-carb tomato sauce

- 1 cup mozzarella cheese, shredded

- 1 cup parmesan cheese, grated

- 1 cup ricotta cheese

- 1 Tablespoon fresh basil leaves, chopped

- 1 Tablespoon fresh oregano, chopped

- 1 Tablespoon paprika

- 1 teaspoon salt

- 1 teaspoon fresh ground black pepper

## Directions:

Grease a baking dish with non-stick cooking spray.

In a bowl, combine the cheeses and herbs.

In a separate bowl, add and season the eggplants with garlic cloves, lemon juice, paprika, salt, and black pepper.

Layer baking dish with eggplant slices, tomato sauce. Sprinkle mixed cheeses. Repeat.

Cover baking dish with aluminum foil.

Add 2 cups of water. Place trivet in Instant Pot. Place dish on trivet.

Close and seal lid. Press Manual switch. Cook at High Pressure for 25 minutes.

When done, naturally release or quickly release pressure. Open the lid with care. Serve.

# Unbelievable Zucchini with Avocado Sauce

**Prep + Cook Time**: 15 minutes

## Ingredients

- 2 pounds of zucchini, chopped

- 2 avocados, chopped

- Juice from 1 lime

- 1 shallot, chopped

- 2 garlic cloves, minced

- 1 cup of water

- 2 Tablespoons coconut oil

- ¼ cup fresh basil, chopped

- 1 teaspoon salt (to taste)

- 1 teaspoon fresh ground black pepper (to taste)

## Directions:

Press Sauté mode on Instant Pot. Heat the coconut oil.

Sauté garlic and shallots for 1 minute. Press Keep Warm/Cancel setting to stop Sauté mode.

Add zucchini, avocado, basil, salt, and black pepper. Stir well. Add the water. Stir well.

Close and seal lid. Press Manual setting. Cook at High Pressure for 5 minutes.

Quick-release or naturally release pressure. Open the lid with care. Stir ingredients.

Allow to cool down or refrigerate overnight.

# To-Die For Curried Cauliflower

**Prep + Cook Time**: 55 minutes

## Ingredients

1 large head of cauliflower

1 medium-sized yellow onion, finely chopped

2 tomatoes, chopped

2 garlic cloves, minced

1 ½ cups of full-fat yogurt

2 tablespoons of curry powder

1 teaspoon of smoked or regular paprika

2 tablespoons of freshly squeezed lemon juice

1 teaspoon of lemon zest

1 teaspoon of sea salt

1 ½ teaspoons of freshly cracked black pepper

½ cup of pine nuts

¼ cup of fresh cilantro, finely chopped

¼ cup of olive oil

4 tablespoons of feta cheese, crumbled.

## Directions:

Preheat your oven to 375 degrees Fahrenheit.

Line a baking sheet with parchment powder.

In a large bowl, add the chopped onion, minced garlic, yogurt, curry powder, paprika, lemon juice, lemon zest, black pepper, and sea salt. Rub the mixture over the head of cauliflower.

Place the cauliflower on the baking sheet and place inside your oven. Bake for 45 minutes or until crispy. Remove and set aside.

In a blender, add the tomatoes and ¼ cup of the pine nuts. Pulse until chunky. Transfer to a bowl.

Add the fresh cilantro, remaining pine nuts, olive oil, and feta cheese. Stir until well combined.

Chop the cauliflower into florets and transfer to a dish. Drizzle with the tomato mixture. Transfer to containers and enjoy!

# Comforting Green Bean Casserole

**Prep + Cook Time**: 45 minutes

## Ingredients

1 pound of green beans, halved

½ cup of almond flour or coconut flour

2 tablespoons of butter

1 cup of mushrooms, chopped

½ medium-sized onions, finely chopped

2 medium shallots, finely chopped

3 garlic cloves, minced

½ cup of homemade low-sodium chicken broth

½ cup of heavy cream

¼ cup of finely grated Parmesan cheese

1 teaspoon of sea salt

1 teaspoon of freshly cracked black pepper

2 tablespoons of avocado oil.

## Directions:

Preheat your oven to 400 degrees Fahrenheit.

In a large pot, add water and bring to a boil over medium-high heat.

Once the water is boiling, add the green beans and cook for 5 minutes.

Once done, drain and transfer the green beans to an ice bath. Allow to cool.

In a bowl, combine the chopped shallots, chopped onions, almond flour, sea salt and black pepper.

In a large pan, heat 2 tablespoons of avocado oil over medium-high heat.

Add the shallot mixture to the pan and cook until golden color.

Once done, transfer the shallot mixture to a plate lined with paper towels.

Return the frying pan to the stove and add 2 tablespoons of butter.

Once the butter has melted, add the minced garlic and chopped mushrooms. Cook for 5 minutes, stirring occasionally.

Add the chicken broth and heavy cream to the pan. Bring to a boil and simmer until thickens.

Stir in the finely grated parmesan cheese and green beans. Stir until well coated. Remove the pan from the heat.

Transfer the mixture to a baking dish and sprinkle with the crispy shallot mixture.

Place the baking dish inside your oven and bake for 15 minutes or until brown on top. Carefully remove the baking dish from your oven and allow to cool. Transfer the casserole to containers and enjoy!

# Asian-Inspired Bok Choy Stir-Fry

**Prep + Cook Time**: 20 minutes

## Ingredients

4 cups of bok choy, chopped

1 cup of shitake mushrooms, sliced

1 red bell pepper, thinly sliced

2 leeks, sliced

4 garlic cloves, minced

2 tablespoons of avocado oil, olive oil, and coconut oil

2 tablespoons of low-sodium coconut aminos

1 teaspoon of fish sauce

½ teaspoon of white pepper

## Directions:

Heat a frying pan with the avocado oil over medium-high heat.

Add the sliced leeks, minced garlic, thinly sliced red bell pepper, shitake mushrooms and cook until lightly softened, stirring occasionally. Add the bok choy and cook for 4 minutes, stirring occasionally.

Add the coconut aminos, fish sauce, and white pepper. Cook for an additional minute.

Divide among containers and enjoy!

# Gentle Sautéed Mustard Greens

**Prep + Cook Time**: 30 minutes

**Ingredients**

2 ½ pounds of mustard greens, chopped

1 tablespoon of olive oil

2 garlic cloves, minced

1 teaspoon of freshly squeezed lemon juice

1 tablespoon of butter

½ teaspoon of sea salt

½ teaspoon of freshly cracked black pepper

**Directions**:

In a large pot, add water. Bring to simmer over medium heat. Add the mustard greens and cover with a lid. Cook for 15 minutes. Once done, drain the collard greens and remove excess liquid. Transfer to a bowl.

Heat a large pan with olive oil and butter over medium-high heat.

Once hot, add the mustard greens, sea salt, black pepper, garlic cloves, and lemon juice. Sauté for 5 minutes, stirring occasionally. Divide the greens amongst containers and enjoy!

# CONCLUSION

I hope the book was was informative and provided you with tons of useful information to help change the rest of your life through each segment of your journey by providing you with the fundamentals of the ketogenic way of living. Each tasty recipe is designed to keep you in ketosis. The first few weeks may be a little stressful but hang in there because it will become easier.

Once you have all of the chief spices and other fixings stocked in your keto kitchen, the following week's shopping list will be much simpler. As a quick reminder, keep these simple tips in mind as you go through your ketogenic journey:

- Drink plenty of water daily and limit the intake of sugar-sweetened beverages.

- It is essential to attempt to use only half of your typical serving of salad dressing or butter.

- Use only fat-free or low-fat condiments.

- Add a serving of vegetables to your dinner and lunch menus.

- Add a serving of fruit as a snack or enjoy with your meal. The skin also contains additional nutrients. Dried and canned fruits are quick and easy to use. However, make sure they don't have added sugar.

- Read the food labels and make choices that keep you in line with ketosis.

- For a snack have some frozen yogurt (fat-free or low-fat), nuts or unsalted pretzels, raw veggies, unsalted-plain popcorn.

- Prepare cut veggies such as bell pepper strips, mixed greens, and carrots. Store them in small baggies for a quick on-the-go healthy choice.

Made in the USA
Columbia, SC
06 May 2020